STRATEGY OF DRUG DESIGN:
A GUIDE TO BIOLOGICAL ACTIVITY

Strategy of Drug Design: A Guide to Biological Activity

WILLIAM P. PURCELL

GEORGE E. BASS

JOHN M. CLAYTON

Department of Molecular and Quantum Biology
College of Pharmacy
University of Tennessee Medical Units, Memphis

A WILEY-INTERSCIENCE PUBLICATION

JOHN WILEY & SONS, New York • London • Sydney • Toronto

Library of Congress Cataloging in Publication Data:

Purcell, William P.
Strategy of Drug Design: A Guide to Biological Activity

"A Wiley-Interscience publication."
1. Structure-activity relationship (Pharmacology)—Mathematical models. I. Bass, George E., joint author. II. Clayton, John M., joint author. III. Title. [DNLM: 1. Biometry. 2. Models, Biologic. 3. Models, Chemical. QH 324 P985m 1973]

QP909.P87 574.8′8 72–13240
ISBN 0–471–70236–6

Printed in the United States of America

10 9 8 7 6 5 4 3 2 1

PREFACE

This book was written to introduce organic chemists, medicinal chemists, pharmacologists, graduate students, and others to the techniques of applying mathematical models to the design of molecules with desired biological activities. It is hoped that the book will be a convenient desk reference for these techniques and serve as a "how-to-do-it" text. It is not intended to be a textbook on physical-organic chemistry, statistics, or quantum chemistry; other books are available which treat these subjects most adequately.

Chapter I introduces the subject, gives an historical review of the development of quantitative structure-activity relationships (QSAR) and presents some justification for the use of these tools in designing a molecule for a specific biological purpose. The rest of the book is devoted to two approaches in QSAR: the Linear Free Energy-Related (LFER) or Extrathermodynamic models (Chapters II-IV), which deal with the correlation of physicochemical properties of a molecule with its biological activity, and the *De Novo* model (Chapters V and VI), which is a statistical approach, independent of physicochemical properties, for ranking substituent group contributions to biological activity.

The section on the LFER models is divided into three chapters: the underlying theory (Chapter II); reference to the applications of the method and tables of hydrophobic, steric, and electronic parameters (Chapter III); and a simple hypothetical step-by-step example of two "real-life" examples (Chapter IV). These three chapters are intended to serve different purposes and may be read independently or simply used as reference sources. In Chapter III, for example, we do not attempt to define and explain the Taft steric parameter (Table 3.2); rather we point out that it is used in the LFER model and give 22 references to it. Chapter IV was written to show the reader how to use the method by guiding him through a simple example. Two examples follow to bring the theory into perspective with real applications.

Chapter V and VI are analogous to the section on the LFER model. The main difference is that much less work has been done using the De Novo model; therefore, the theory is introduced in a short chapter followed by a detailed hypothetical example and two real examples in Chapter VI.

The reader may find some sections written like a review article and some sections written like a detailed teaching text. Our objectives are such that this style is intentional.

On a slightly philosophical note, we might add that we recognize that this approach does not represent a panacea to drug design and that biological systems are not ready to lie quietly while we dissect and probe with neat mathematical models and laws of physics. We do see tremendous potential in the application of mathematics, physics, and chemistry (including advances in computer technology) to problems of biological interest; further, we can envision a day when the biological activity data become more quantitative and the models become more refined and meaningful, and when one will be able to predict rather accurately the biological activity of a molecule before it is even synthesized.

William P. Purcell

Memphis, Tennessee
November 1972

CONTENTS

STRATEGY OF DRUG DESIGN:
A GUIDE TO BIOLOGICAL ACTIVITY

CHAPTER I

INTRODUCTION

The planning and architectural concepts underlying the selection of a molecule which would be a promising candidate as a useful therapeutic agent carry the label "drug design." This same activity, however, is being applied to the search for more effective herbicides, pesticides, and the like, and it is in this broad sense that structure-activity relationships are considered here. Even though the last 100 years produced more examples of attempts to correlate changes in molecular structure with changes in drug-like activities, the methodology is perfectly general and the spectrum of disciplines associated with the research continues to widen.

Until about the middle of the twentieth century, most of the correlation studies were empirical and qualitative, but more recent work shows a bold effort to make the correlations quantitative via mathematical models with predictive capabilities. Paralleling the growth of interest in quantitative structure-activity relationship (QSAR) studies, there has been improvement in the techniques for isolating the physicochemical factors associated with a particular biological mechanism. The ultimate goal is obvious: to predict the biological activity of a molecule prior to evaluation or even synthesis in order to reduce the costly and time-consuming synthetic work and biological screening. From another point of view, it is hoped that the application of QSAR studies will elucidate the mechanism of the interaction of a given molecule with a biological system.

Around 1865-1870, Crum-Brown and Fraser published what might be considered the first structure-activity relationship study of molecules of pharmacological interest (1). They showed that the gradual chemical modification in the molecular structure of a series of poisons produced some important differences in their actions. In a study of such compounds as strychnine, brucine, thebain, codeine, morphine, and nicotine, they observed distinct changes in the degree of activity paralleling somewhat minor changes in chemical structures (1,2). With their observations having been further substantiated by studies on atropine and conine, Crum-Brown and Fraser postulated that the physiological action, Φ, of a molecule is some function of its chemical constitution, C (1.1).

$$\Phi = f(C) \tag{1.1}$$

They concurred that the only reason that such a correlation was not strictly mathematical was their inability to express the terms $\Delta C, \Phi$, and $\Phi + \Delta\Phi$ quantitatively as required for such a treatment. ΔC represents a defined change in chemical constitution and $\Delta\Phi$ symbolizes a corresponding incremental change in biological activity (1,2).

Studying the toxicities of a variety of ethers, alcohols, aldehydes, and ketones, Richet concluded in 1893 that their degree of activity was inversely related to their water solubility (3). This postulate, known as Richet's rule, was the first published experimental evidence of Crum-Brown and Fraser's theory. At the turn of the twentieth century Meyer and Overton applied Richet's work quite extensively to other series of liquid compounds (4-7). Studying the lipid solubility of congeners that possessed narcotic activity, they observed that most organic compounds foreign to the body penetrate tissue cells as though the membranes were lipid in nature. They further noted that passage across these barriers and the resulting narcotic activity paralleled their oil-water partitioning properties. This treatment was theorized to simulate the *in vivo* situation of a drug's partitioning between an aqueous exobiophase and a lipophilic receptor site. This is the first reported correlation between partition coefficients and biological activity.

Further investigations of the relationship between other physicochemical properties of molecules and their elicited biological responses were made by Traube in 1904 (8). In studies of a variety of narcotic agents he observed a linear relationship between the surface tensions of the compounds and their narcotic activity. At approximately the same time Fühner attempted the quantitative correlation between the narcotic action of a diverse group of molecules with the number of carbon atoms in the compound (9-11). He demonstrated that the decrease in the molecular concentration necessary to produce a defined response over the homologous series followed a geometric progression ($1:3:3^2:3^3 \ldots$) corresponding to an increase in the number of carbon atoms (11). Moore used another physicochemical parameter in structure-activity studies in 1917 (12,13). As a result of a series of experiments with a large number of different chemicals, he observed that the toxicity to insects of the vapor of an organic compound is correlated directly with its volatility or boiling point (12-15). Later studies based on Traube's work led Warburg in 1921 to postulate a mechanism of narcotic action for these compounds (16).

A very important second step in QSAR was made by Ferguson in 1939 when he demonstrated an interrelationship among much of the earlier work (17). Using Equations 1.2 and 1.3,

$$C_r = kS_r^{1/n} \tag{1.2}$$

$$C_r = kp_r^{1/n} \tag{1.3}$$

he was able to calculate the toxic concentrations, C, of a series of compounds from solubility and vapor pressure data. In equations 1.2 and 1.3, C_r is the toxic concentration of the _r_th member of the series, S_r is its solubility in moles per liter, p_r is its vapor pressure, and k and n are constants with n always greater than one. From this study, a generalized equation (1.4) was postulated to describe the biological responses of several congeneric series (17-19):

$$C_i = kA_i^m \tag{1.4}$$

C_i is the concentration of the _i_th congener necessary to elicit a defined response, A_i is a physicochemical or descriptive parameter for the compound (e.g., partition coefficient, number of carbon atoms in a side chain, solubility, vapor pressure, etc.), and K and m are constants for the series. The negative logarithm of Equation 1.4 becomes Equation 1.5 which is more useful in QSAR studies:

$$-\log C_i = -\log k - m \log A_i \tag{1.5}$$

Incorporating the negative signs into constants k and m (i.e., by redefining k = -log k and m = -n), Equation 1.5 becomes the somewhat more familiar Equation 1.6:

$$\log 1/C_i = k + m \log A_i \tag{1.6}$$

Further correlations between physicochemical parameters and biological activity made by McGowan in 1951 (20-22). In the study of the physical toxicity of a variety of chemicals to different biological systems, he found that Equation 1.7 gave excellent correlations for the diverse systems (20):

$$\log C = (7.7 + S) + (4 \times 10^{23})p - 0.036\ [P] \tag{1.7}$$

In equation 1.7, C is the toxic concentration of vapor of the chemical in parts per million, S is a sensitivity factor based upon varying sensitivity of different biological systems to a series of compounds, p is the polarizability of the gas or vapor, and [P] represents the molecular volume or parachor of the chemical. His study led him to postulate that the biophase concerned is either very similar or identical in all organisms studied. Other studies by McGowan (21-24) extended his correlation studies to a variety of liquids and solutions with apparent success. These studies included the incorporation of partition coefficient, boiling point, and interaction terms into the equations.

Perhaps one of the most important contributions to the development of QSAR models was reported in 1956 by Bruice, Kharasch, and Winzler (25). Their empirical, mathematical model, which marked the beginning of studies which were to proliferate in the 1960s, was applied to the correlation of thyroxine-like activities of a series of congeners with the sum of constants assigned to different substituents on the molecules. Using Equation 1.8, they obtained excellent correlations between calculated and observed biological activities:

$$\log \%\ \text{thyroxine-like activity} = K\Sigma f + c \tag{1.8}$$

In Equation 1.8, $\Sigma f = (f_X + f_{X'} + f_{OR'})$, where f_X, $f_{X'}$, and $f_{OR'}$ are entirely empirical and were selected by a method similar to that of Hammett for the evaluation of sigma constants, and c is a constant. Subscripts X, X' and OR' represent substituent positions of the molecules of interest (15).

An important contribution which will be treated in detail in Chapters V and VI is the development of a QSAR model by Free and Wilson in 1964 (26). It is an example of what we will categorize as the "*de novo*" model. They defined the biological response (BR) as equal to the sum of the contributions to the activity of the substituent groups plus the overall average activity (μ) which might be attributed to the activity contribution of the parent structure (Equation 1.9) (26):

$$BR = \Sigma \text{ (substituent group contributions)} + \mu \quad (1.9)$$

The main purpose of this treatment is to rank the biological activities of the substituent groups while noting possible structure-activity relationships and to predict the compounds of the series not tested, and possibly not synthesized, which would have the greatest potential for further investigation. The major limitation of the method lies in the fact that the activity contributions of the substituents must be additive.

At approximately the same time as Free and Wilson's work, Kopecký, Boćek, and Vlachová introduced a similar mathematical QSAR model (27, 28). Based upon a multiplicative as well as an additive model, their method employed four basic equations (1.10-1.13):

$$BA = a_x - a_y \quad (1.10)$$

$$BA = b_x b_y \quad (1.11)$$

$$BA = c_x + c_y - d_x d_y \quad (1.12)$$

$$BA = c_x + c_y + d_x d_y \quad (1.13)$$

in which a, b, c, and d represent the substituent contributions to the total activities of the compounds while the subscripts x and y denote the substituent positions on the parent molecule, and BA represents the total biological activity for the molecule. Testing these equations for the expression of the quantitative difference between the log LD_{50} (LD_{50} = concentration necessary to kill 50% of the population) values of *para*- (27) and *meta*- (28) disubstituted benzenes and benzene, they found that neither the additive model (1.10), the multiplicative model (1.11), nor the combined difference expression (1.12) described the biological activity adequately. The combined summation expression (1.13), however, gave a statistically significant correlation between substituent activity and total biological activity for both the *meta*- (28) and *para*- (27) disubstituted congeners.

At the same time as the postulation and first application of the mathematical model of QSAR were being made, the development of another type of approach, the linear free energy-related (LFER) model (now often called extrathermodynamic), was introduced (29). With the Hammett equation (30, 31) for the hydrolysis rates of benzoic acid derivatives (Equation 1.14) as a basis, i.e.,

$$\log (k_X/k_H) = \rho\sigma \tag{1.14}$$

several investigators have attempted quantitative correlations between physicochemical properties of molecules and their biological responses (32, 33). In Equation 1.14, k_X and k_H are the equilibrium constants for the reactions of substituted and unsubstituted compounds, respectively, σ is a constant which is dependent entirely on the nature and position of the substituent, and ρ is a constant dependent on the type and conditions of the reaction as well as the nature of the compounds (31). When Equation 1.14 is solved for log k_X, i.e.,

$$\log k_X = \rho\sigma + \log k_H \tag{1.15}$$

the Hammett equation clearly illustrates the linear relationship between the substituent constant σ and the logarithm of the reactivity of the compound (k_X) (33, 34). Since the logarithm of an equilibrium constant is proportional to the change in Gibbs free energy (35), i.e.,

$$\Delta G° = -RT \ln k \tag{1.16}$$

Equation 1.15 and others like it are said to be "free energy-related" (34); therefore, this phrase will be used to include all models of this type. Since Hansch pioneered the approach, it is often called the Hansch model. In Equation 1.16, $\Delta G°$ is the change in Gibbs free energy, R is the ideal gas constant, T is the absolute temperature, and k is the equilibrium constant for the reaction. From about 1952 to 1966 several investigators have applied this Hammet LFER equation to many biological systems; however, they met with very limited degrees of success (32, 36-43). With a number of these applications as a basis, in 1962 Hansen proposed a "biological Hammett equation" (44):

$$-\log (H\sigma)_q + \log (Ho)_q = \rho\sigma \tag{1.17}$$

Using Equation 1.17 in which $(H\sigma)_q$ and $(Ho)_q$ are the concentrations of the inhibitor of the substituted and parent compound, respectively, in a Hammett series necessary to give a defined percentage response q, while ρ and σ are the Hammett constants, Hansen was able to correlate successfully bacterial growth inhibition of several series of compounds with their Hammett sigma (σ) constants. In spite of its very restrictive set of conditions, however, the "biological Hammett equation" has met with only limited success (44).

The application of the Hammett equation was extended by Zahradník and co-workers to correlate other physicochemical parameters of homologous series of compounds with their biological activities (45). The basis of their correlations was Equation 1.18:

$$\log (\tau_i/\tau_{et}) = \alpha\beta \tag{1.18}$$

where τ_i and τ_{et} are the molar concentrations of the *i*th congener and ethyl derivative, respectively, of an homologous series necessary to elicit a defined biological response, α is a constant which is dependent upon the nature of the series of compounds and the biological system, and β is a physicochemical parameter which is dependent upon the particular substituent group. Different β values (including Hammett and Taft constants) have been used on several homologous series of compounds in various biological systems (45-48). Again, the use of a single parameter, however, has given correlations of limited significance.

Recognizing the physicochemical nature of biological reactions and realizing, as did Overton and others several years prior to 1965 (49, 50), the importance of partitioning in a drug's transport to its ultimate site of action, Hansch and co-workers expanded the Hammett LFER expression to include additional physicochemical parameters (51-53). Following the approach used by Taft (54) in the linear combination of two physicochemical constants, they derived the ρ-σ-π equation (1.19) for the correlation of biological activity with molecular structure (51):

$$\log (1/C) = k_1\pi + \rho\sigma + k_2 \tag{1.19}$$

In this equation C represents the molar concentration of a congener in the series necessary to elicit a defined biological response, π is the substituent partitioning parameter defined as the difference between the logarithms of the octanol/water partition coefficients of the substituted and unsubstituted parent compounds in the series (55), σ is the Hammett substituent constant, and k_1, ρ, and k_2 are constants for the series generated by regression analysis of the data. Although all of these terms are free energy-related and approximate true thermodynamic constants, the expression is said to be "extrathermodynamic" since the parameters are used in systems other than those similar to the systems in which they were determined (51,56).

After meeting with a great deal of success in correlating the structure-activity data from hundreds of systems (57,58), this basic equation has been modified by the addition or substitution of a variety of parameters in attempts to find better correlations. One of the foremost modifications of this basic equation has been Hansch's postulate that the biological response to a drug is parabolically rather than linearly related to its partitioning properties. This resulted in the inclusion of the π^2 term (52,53,59) as shown in Equation 1.20 (in which k is also a constant generated by the regression analysis):

$$\log (1/C) = k\pi^2 + k_1\pi + \rho\sigma + k_2 \qquad (1.20)$$

Although it may seem that the parameters in Equation 1.20 are somewhat arbitrary and highly empirical, it can be shown that these variables can be derived from first principles if one assumes a random walk process by which a drug reaches its site of action (52).

An important advantage of this extrathermodynamic or LFER approach lies in its flexibility to modification by incorporation or deletion of physicochemical parameters to describe more adequately a particular biological phenomenon. For example, it has been used by Hansch and Deutsch to aid in the elucidation of the mechanism of drug action at the submolecular level by determination of the relative importance of each type of parameter in describing the biological response (60). Of course, the quantitative nature of the LFER model is limited by the accuracy of the biological data (as are all QSAR models), as well as by the accuracy of the experimental physicochemical parameters and their applicability to systems somewhat unrelated to those in which they were determined.

In addition to these attempts at QSAR model building, a theoretical, quantum chemical approach has been applied to the study of chemical compounds of biological interest (61,62,33). Since 1950, the Pullmans have made major contributions in the application of quantum chemistry to biological phenomena (63-66). Their work on the possible mechanism of chemical carcinogenesis in terms of quantum mechanical properties as well as calculations on the nucleic acid constituents has laid much of the foundation for the increasing interest in quantum biology (63-66). At a somewhat more fundamental level, Löwdin has also been a pioneer in the application of quantum mechanics to the problems of biological and biochemical interest (67). He has proposed a mechanism of deoxyribonucleic acid (DNA) replication based on his theoretical calculations.

Other related work appeared in 1965 when Neely published an example of the utility of molecular orbital theory in biological activity correlation studies (68). He illustrated the use of quantum chemical calculations as an aid in the correlation of the submolecular structure of selected organophosphates and carbamates with their cholinesterase inhibitory potencies (68). Kier has been another pioneer in the utilization of these techniques to postulate the nature of several biological receptors. Through quantum mechanical calculations, he has predicted the preferred conformations of isolated molecules of biological interest and has related their lowest energy conformations to the nature of their receptors (69-75).

These methods have been used in the physicochemical approach to drug design. Applying the mathematical model of Free and Wilson (26), Beasley and Purcell have given the first example of a successful prediction of the activity of a compound three years prior to its synthesis (76). In 1965 they reported the calculated butyrylcholinesterase inhibitory potency of 1-decyl-3-(N-ethyl-N-methylcarbamoyl)piperidine hydrobromide (77). Three years later this compound was synthesized and evaluated biochemically. The observed and predicted response values agreed within the limits of experimental error (76). Ban and Fujita also obtained excellent correlations between calculated and observed response values in the study of the norepinephrine uptake inhibition of selected sympathomimetic amines (78).

More efforts, however, have been concerned with the attempts to correlate molecular structure and biological activity using physicochemical parameters in modification of the LFER expressions (79-83). Although the basic transport and electronic parameters are usually retained, the application of several parameters other than π and σ

has been studied. For example, Hansch and co-workers have obtained excellent correlations using log P, where P is the partition coefficient of the entire compound, in place of the summation of the substituent parameters π (84,85). Although partitioning systems other than that of octanol/water have been used for the *in vitro* simulation of the *in vivo* situation, very little improvement, if any, has been shown in the correlations using other systems (86,87). Others have obtained excellent correlations by use of the chromatographic parameter R_M to approximate the transport process (88-93).

Further extensive variation in parameters has been reported in the approximation of the electronic substituent parameters. In addition to the widely used Hammett σ parameter for aromatic systems, many investigators have applied the Taft σ^* parameter to aliphatic systems with varying degrees of success (29,54,56,79,83,94,95). McFarland has suggested the use of group dipole moments, μ, and the electronic polarizability parameter α in addition to σ values in order to explain the electronic factors involved in drug-receptor interactions (96,97). He has obtained excellent correlations between the inhibitory rate constants of *E. coli* and the properties of certain chloramphenicol analogs using these parameters (Equation 1.21) (96):

$$\log (1/C) = k_1\pi^2 + k_2\pi + k_3\sigma + k_4\mu + k_5\alpha + k_6 \quad (1.21)$$

More recently he has given an extensive derivation of the theoretical basis for the inclusion of these parameters; he also treated the parabolic relationship between drug potency and hydrophobicity (97).

In other applications of the method, Clayton and Purcell have illustrated the predictive utility of such expressions in a study of selected butyrylcholinesterase inhibitors (94). They obtained quantitative correlations between the calculated and observed biological activities by using Taft σ^* substituent parameters, amide group dipole moments and total dipole moment values, in addition to substituent partitioning parameters (94). Hansch and co-workers have used Taft steric parameters (E_s) (56) and pK_a values to achieve significant correlations (84). E_s has recently been shown to be quantitatively related to van der Waal's radii for symmetrical toplike substituents (98) while pK_a values have been used as a measure of the electron density distributions (99). Fukuto and co-workers have combined E_s and σ^* parameters in a physicochemical approach to elucidating the mode of action of organophosphorous insecticides (95).

Garrett et al. have used modified Hammett substituent constants (100) to describe the bacteriostatic activities of a series of sulfanilamides (101). The homolytic substituent constants E_R of Yamamoto and Otsu (102) were applied by Hansch to analyze the activity of selected chloramphenicol derivatives (103). The results of his study led to the hypothesis of a free-radical mechanism of chloramphenicol action. Other estimates of the electronic factors involved in drug-receptor interactions have been used by Sasaki and Suzuki (104). They approached the problem by using substituent measures of π-electron charge density distributions (σ_I and σ_π) (105) to illustrate the dependence of partition coefficients and biological activity on molecular electronic conditions (104).

In addition to these, other thermodynamic substituent constants have been investigated (33,79,106). For example, Ostrenga has considered molar attraction constants (107, 108) and Turner and Battershell have correlated chemical reactivities, vapor pressures, and partition coefficients of a series of isophthalonitriles with their fungicidal properties (109).

Jones and co-workers have used regression analysis to study the effects of field constants and resonance parameters (110) of some carbamate derivatives on their penetration and detoxication with some success (111). Similar studies have been made by Fukuto and co-workers using selected oximes and their anti-cholinesterase activities (112). Kakeya et al. have used chemical shifts and valence force constants in addition to other thermodynamic parameters in the structure-activity study of a series of sulfonamide carbonic anhydrase inhibitors (113).

The combination of quantum mechanical calculations and the LFER model presents a wider view in drug activity studies; a variety of indices obtained from the quantum chemical calculations have been utilized in these correlations (79,83,114-116). For example, Neely and co-workers have obtained excellent correlations between the energy of the highest occupied molecular orbital (HOMO), a relative measure of the ability of a molecule to donate an electron to an acceptor molecule, of a series of imidazolines and their analgetic potencies (117).

In an analysis of the linear free energy relationship in drug-receptor interactions, Cammarata has shown a theoretical interpretation of substituent constants in a biological context (118,119). He has separated the free energy change occurring in a reaction into its electronic, desolvation, and steric components; defined each in terms of contributions made to it; and approximated these contributions with quantum mechanical indices (120, 121). Using atomic orbital coefficients and total electronic charge on certain portions of the molecule, Cammarata has obtained excellent correlations between quantum mechanical indices and sulfanilamide activity (122). He has also suggested the use of π-electrophilic and nucleophilic superdelocalizabilities and energy level differences to interpret drug-receptor interactions. When this approach was applied to selected cholinesterase inhibitors, he obtained very good correlations (123). Wohl has combined several quantum mechanical parameters determined from the Extended Hückel Theory in a LFER study of the biological potencies and electronic structures of several benzothiadiazine derivatives. The quantitative correlation that he obtained led to certain postulations concerning the centers of the molecules which are most responsible for the biological responses due to their electronic properties (115,116).

Hermann et al. have obtained good correlations between the relative substrate efficiencies of some acetophenones toward rabbit kidney reductase and selected quantum mechanical parameters (124). The substituent indices were derived from electron density calculations and energy differences between ground and incipient transition states (124). In the study of the DNA intercalation by chloroquine derivatives, Bass et al. (125) calculated the sigma-electron charge distributions and used these in addition to other substituent parameters to investigate a mechanism proposed by O'Brien and Hahn (126) for antimalarial activity. The derivation of and rationale behind the inclusion of this term into the Hansch equation were also given (125).

It may appear that the various structure-activity models and parameters are not truly as independent as they are presented here. Certainly this suspicion is justified. Singer and Purcell have evaluated the interrelationships among the quantitative structure-activity models and have illustrated their similarities (127). Also, the parameters used in these models cannot be completely independent of one another. In most of the literature, the investigators have merely attempted to find those parameters which alone or in combination best describe the biological activity. Along these lines, Leo et al. have reported a comparison of the parameters currently used in studies of this type (86).

Apart from their use in LFER equations, quantum mechanical calculations have been used in other ways in drug design studies. Nagy and Nador have found that the central exciting effect of amphetamines increases with a decrease of the negative charge, as determined by quantum mechanical methods, on the second carbon of the benzene ring (128). Corcodano has calculated the ring carbon reactivity indices of some phenylacetic acid derivatives and has shown that this parameter correlates well with their auxinic activities (129). Using the Hückel molecular orbital method, Mainster and Memory have proposed that superdelocalizability may be used in the characterization of chemical carcinogens (130).

In other studies, Purcell and Sundaram have used the sum of the energy of the highest occupied molecular orbital (HOMO) and that of the lowest empty molecular orbital (LEMO) as a measure of molecular electronegativity when applied to quinolinemethanol antimalarials (131). Sharpless and Greenblatt have found that electron density, LEMO, and pK_a values correlate well with the acridine toxicities to various microorganisms (132). These correlations have led to their postulation of a mechanism of action. In a final example, Andrews has used quantum chemical methods to calculate the dipole moments of a series of anticonvulsant drugs and related compounds (133). These calculations suggest a mechanism of action for these drugs different from that which had been proposed previously (134).

One additional area of increasing interest in the physicochemical approach to drug design is the use of instrumental methods, particularly nuclear magnetic resonance (nmr). Pioneered by Jardetzky and co-workers (135,136), the use of nmr in studies of drug-receptor interactions at the molecular level is showing great promise. This technique is used primarily to follow the change effected in the relaxation rates of the protons of a small molecule upon binding to a macromolecule by observing differential peak broadening of its nmr spectrum. In addition, changes in the chemical shift of the nmr spectrum of the small molecule have been used to investigate substrate-receptor interactions. Thus far, nmr has been successfully applied to the study of enzyme-substrate interactions (137,138), enzyme-coenzyme interactions (139), and enzyme-inhibitor interactions (140, 138). Although the literature is beginning to show numerous _in vitro_ examples of the utility of nmr in this area, one recent application has used the intact cellular system (141). In this study, Fischer and Jost have directly observed the interaction of epinephrine with its receptor site in the mouse liver cell and have been able to postulate the nature of the interaction (141).

From this introduction, it should be apparent that advances have been and are being made in the physicochemical approaches to drug design. Although progress has been slow in developing QSAR, because of the complexity of the biological systems underlying an observable response from a drug, and although there is no promise that these techniques offer a panacea in drug design, there is great potential in "dissecting the role of the important molecular forces at work which yield different biological responses in the series of congeners" (142) and in using physicochemical methods for selecting promising molecules for synthesis and evaluation.

As in virtually all areas of scientific advancement, the various areas of endeavor are at different levels of sophistication. For example, one knows more about the molecular structure of an isolated molecule from instrumental analyses than about the specific interaction of this molecule with a complicated biological system. Illustrating this condition in another way, one could say that the level of sophistication of handling simultaneous equations is greater than the understanding of a parameter from pharmacological testing. It is important, however, to recognize that certain areas will lag behind others as one attempts more rigorous interpretations in interactions between molecules and biological systems. In the authors opinion, this does not mean that work should stop in one area in order for the level of sophistication to "catch up" in another area. Rather, the entire activity should move along without one's becoming preoccupied with the imbalance of the levels of development of the areas of activity. For example, it is most fortunate that the postulation of the Schrödinger equation (143) did not "wait" for the invention of high-speed digital computers, which could give practical application to its solution. This analogy holds for drug design. That is, one should continue efforts to put structure-activity relationships on a quantitative level, even though there are limitations in the biological activity data and bold approximations in the mathematical models. As long as the investigators are aware of these limitations and approximations, it seems perfectly appropriate to continue to improve the data and refine the models.

REFERENCES

1. A. Crum-Brown and T. Fraser, Trans. Roy. Soc. Edinburgh 25, 151 (1868-1869).
2. A Crum-Brown and T. R. Fraser, Trans. Roy. Soc. Edinburgh 25, 693 (1868-1869).
3. M. C. Richet, C. R. Soc. Biol. 45, 775 (1893).
4. H. Meyer, Arch. Exptl. Pathol. Pharmakol. 42, 109 (1899).
5. E. Overton, Z. Physikol. Chem. 22, 189 (1897).
6. E. Overton, Vierteljahresschr. Naturforsch. Ges. Zuerich 44, 88 (1899).
7. E. Overton, Studien uber die Narkose, p. 45, Fischer, Jena, Germany, 1901.
8. J. Traube, Arch. Ges Physiol. (Pflügers) 105, 541 (1904).
9. H. Fühner, Arch. Exptl. Pathol. Pharmakol. 51, 1 (1904).
10. H. Fühner, Arch. Exptl. Pathol. Pharmakol. 52, 69 (1904).
11. H. Fühner and E. Weubauer, Arch. Exptl. Pathol. Pharmakol. 56, 333 (1907).
12. W. Moore, J. Agr. Res. 9, 371 (1917).
13. W. Moore, J. Agr. Res. 10, 365 (1917).
14. W. Moore and S. A. Graham, J. Agr. Res. 13, 523 (1918).
15. W. Moore, Science 49, 572 (1919).
16. O. Warburg, Biochem. Z. 119, 134 (1921).
17. J. Ferguson, Proc. Roy. Soc., Ser. B. 127, 387 (1939).
18. J. Ferguson, Mechanisme de la Narcose, p. 25, Centre National de la Recherche Scientifique, Paris, 1951.
19. J. Ferguson and H. Pirie, Ann. Appl. Biol. 35, 532 (1948).
20. J. C. McGowan, J. Appl. Chem. (London) 1, S120 (1951).
21. J. C. McGowan, J. Appl. Chem. (London) 4, 41 (1954).
22. J. C. McGowan, Nature 200, 1317 (1963).
23. J. C. McGowan, P. N. Atkinson, and L. H. Ruddle, J. Appl. Chem. 16, 19 (1966).
24. J. C. McGowan, J. Appl. Chem. 16, 103 (1966).
25. T. C. Bruice, N. Kharasch, and R. J. Winzler, Arch. Biochem. Biophys. 62, 305 (1956).
26. S. M. Free, Jr., and J. W. Wilson, J. Med. Chem. 7, 395 (1964).

27. K. Bocek, J. Kopecký, M. Krivucová, and D. Vlachová, Experientia 20, 667 (1964).
28. J. Kopecký, K. Bocek, and D. Vlachová, Nature 207, 981 (1965).
29. C. Hansch, in Drug Design, Vol. I, E. J. Ariens, Ed., pp. 271-342, Academic Press, New York, 1971.
30. L. P. Hammett, Chem. Rev. 17, 125 (1935).
31. L. P. Hammett, Physical Organic Chemistry, 1st ed., pp. 184-199, McGraw-Hill, New York, 1940.
32. W. N. Aldridge and A. N. Davison, Biochem. J. 51, 62 (1952).
33. W. P. Purcell, J. A. Singer, K. Sundaram, and G. L. Parks, in Medicinal Chemistry, 3rd ed., A. Burger, Ed., Chapter 10, John Wiley and Sons, Inc., New York, 1970.
34. P. R. Wells, Linear Free Energy Relationships, Academic Press, London, 1968.
35. I. M. Klotz, Chemical Thermodynamics, p. 278, Prentice-Hall, Englewood Cliffs, N. J., 1950.
36. M. L. Bender and K. Nakamura, J. Amer. Chem. Soc. 8[illegible] 2577 (1962).
37. C. H. Blomquist, Acta Chem. Scand. 20, 1747 (1966).
38. R. L. Nath and N. K. Ghosh, Enzymologia 26, 297 (1963).
39. A. H. Neims, D. C. DeLuca, and L. Hellerman, Biochemistry 5, 203 (1966).
40. W. E. Omerod, Biochem. J. 54, 701 (1953).
41. D. G. O'Sullivan and P. W. Sadler, Arch. Biochem. Biophys. 66, 243 (1957).
42. W. F. Sager and P. C. Parks, Proc. Nat. Acad. Sci. U.S. 52, 408 (1964).
43. J. K. Seydel, Mol. Pharmacol. 2, 259 (1966).
44. O. R. Hansen, Acta Chem. Scand. 16, 1593 (1962).
45. R. Zahradník and M. Chvapil, Experientia 16, 511 (1960).
46. M. Chvapil, R. Zahradník, and B. Cmuchalová, Arch. Int. Pharmacodyn. Ther. 135, 330 (1962).
47. R. Zahradník, Arch. Int. Pharmacodyn. Ther. 135, 311 (1962).
48. R. Zahradník, Experientia 18, 534 (1962).
49. R. Collander, Trans. Faraday Soc. 33, 985 (1937).
50. R. Collander, Physio. Plant. 7, 420 (1954).
51. C. Hansch, Acc. Chem. Res. 2, 232 (1969).
52. C. Hansch and T. Fujita, J. Amer. Chem. Soc. 86, 1616 (1964).
53. C. Hansch, R. M. Muir, T. Fujita, P. P. Maloney, F. Geiger, and M. Streich, J. Amer. Chem. Soc. 85, 2817 (1963).

54. R. W. Taft, in Steric Effects in Organic Chemistry, M. S. Newman, Ed., p. 556, John Wiley and Sons, Inc., New York, 1956.
55. T. Fujita, J. Iwasa, and C. Hansch, J. Amer. Chem. Soc. 86, 5175 (1964).
56. J. E. Leffler and E. Grunwald, Rates and Equilibria of Organic Reactions, John Wiley and Sons, Inc., New York, 1963.
57. C. Hansch, in Proceedings of the 3rd International Pharmacological Meeting, July 24-30, 1966, Vol. 7, pp. 141-167, Pergamon Press, New York, 1968.
58. C. Hansch and A. R. Steward, J. Med. Chem. 7, 691 (1964).
59. C. Hansch, A. R. Steward, S. M. Anderson, and D. Bentley, J. Med. Chem. 11, 1 (1968).
60. C. Hansch and E. W. Deutsch, J. Med. Chem. 8, 705 (1965).
61. L. B. Kier, Ed., Molecular Orbital Studies in Chemical Pharmacology, Springer-Verlag, New York, 1970.
62. W. B. Neely, Mol. Pharmacol. 3, 108 (1967).
63. A. Pullman and B. Pullman, in Physico-chemical Mechanisms of Carcinogenesis, the Jerusalem Symposia on Quantum Chemistry and Biochemistry, I, p. 9, The Israel Academy of Sciences and Humanities, Jerusalem, 1969.
64. B. Pullman, in Electronic Aspects of Biochemistry, B. Pullman, Ed., p. 559, Academic Press, New York, 1964.
65. B. Pullman and A. Pullman, Quantum Biochemistry, Inter-Science Publishers, New York, 1963.
66. B. Pullman, A. Pullman, R. Umans, and B. Maigret in Physico-chemical Mechanisms of Carcinogenesis, The Jerusalem Symposia on Quantum Chemistry and Biochemistry, I, p. 325, The Israel Academy of Sciences and Humanities, Jerusalem, 1969.
67. P. O. Löwdin, in Electronic Aspects of Biochemistry, B. Pullman, Ed., p. 167, Academic Press, New York, 1964.
68. W. B. Neely, Mol. Pharmacol. 1, 137 (1965).
69. L. B. Kier, J. Med. Chem. 11, 441 (1968).
70. L. B. Kier, J. Med. Chem. 11, 915 (1968).
71. L. B. Kier, J. Pharm. Sci. 57, 1188 (1968).
72. L. B. Kier, J. Pharmacol. Exp. Ther. 164, 75 (1968).
73. L. B. Kier, J. Pharm. Pharmacol. 21, 93 (1969).
74. L. B. Kier, J. Pharm. Sci. 59, 112 (1970).
75. L. B. Kier, in Fundamental Concepts in Drug-Receptor Interactions, J. F. Danielli, J. F. Moran, and D. J. Triggle, Eds., p. 15, Academic Press, New York, 1970.

76. J. G. Beasley and W. P. Purcell, Biochim. Biophys. Acta 178, 175 (1969).
77. W. P. Purcell, Biochim. Biophys. Acta 105, 201 (1965).
78. T. Ban and T. Fujita, J. Med. Chem. 12, 353 (1969).
79. J. M. Clayton, O. E. Millner, Jr., and W. P. Purcell, Ann. Rept. Med. Chem., 1969, 285 (1970).
80. C. Hansch, Ann. Rept. Med. Chem., 1966, 347 (1967).
81. C. Hansch, Ann. Rept. Med. Chem., 1967, 348 (1968).
82. C. Hansch, E. W. Deutsch, and R. N. Smith, J. Amer. Chem. Soc. 87, 2738 (1965).
83. W. P. Purcell and J. M. Clayton, Ann. Rept. Med. Chem., 1968, 314 (1969).
84. C. Hansch, E. J. Lien, and F. Helmer, Arch. Biochem Biophys. 128, 319 (1968).
85. E. J. Lien and C. Hansch, J. Pharm. Sci. 57, 1027 (1968).
86. A. Leo, C. Hansch, and C. Church, J. Med. Chem. 12, 766 (1969).
87. E. J. Lien, J. Agr. Food Chem. 17, 1265 (1969).
88. L. S. Bark and R. J. T. Graham, J. Chromatogr. 23, 417 (1966).
89. G. L. Biagi, A. M. Barbaro, M. F. Gamba, and M. C. Guerra, J. Chromatogr. 41, 371 (1969).
90. G. L. Biagi, M. C. Guerra, A. M. Barbaro, and M. F. Gamba, J. Med. Chem. 13, 511 (1970).
91. C. B. C. Boyce and B. V. Milborrow, Nature 208, 537 (1965).
92. J. Iwasa, T. Fujita, and C. Hansch, J. Med. Chem. 8 150 (1965).
93. E. Soczewiński and M. Bieganowska, J. Chromatogr. 40, 431 (1969).
94. J. M. Clayton and W. P. Purcell, J. Med. Chem. 12, 1087 (1969).
95. T. R. Fukuto, in Residue Reviews, F. A. Gunther, Ed., p. 327, Springer-Verlag, New York, 1969.
96. J. W. McFarland, J. Med. Chem. 13, 1192 (1970).
97. J. W. McFarland, Progress in Drug Research 15, 123 (1971).
98. C. Hansch, J. Org. Chem. 35, 620 (1970).
99. E. V. Brown and W. H. Kipp, Cancer Res. 29, 1341 (1969).
100. M. Yoshioka, K. Hamamoto, and T. Kubota, Bull. Chem Soc. Jap. 35, 1723 (1962).
101. E. R. Garrett, J. B. Mielck, J. K. Seydel, and H. J Kessler, J. Med. Chem. 12, 740 (1969).
102. T. Yamamoto and T. Otsu, Chem. Ind. (London), 787 (1967).

103. C. Hansch, E. Kutter, and A. Leo, J. Med. Chem. 12, 746 (1969).
104. Y. Sasaki and M. Suzuki, Chem. Pharm. Bull. (Tokyo) 17, 1596 (1969).
105. Y. Yukawa and Y. Tsuno, J. Chem. Soc. Jap. (Pure Chemistry Section) 86, 873 (1965).
106. W. B. Neely, W. E. Allison, W. B. Crummett, K. Kauer, and W. Reifshneider, J. Agr. Food Chem. 18, 45 (1970).
107. J. A. Ostrenga, J. Med. Chem. 12, 349 (1969).
108. J. A. Ostrenga and C. Steinmetz, J. Pharm. Sci. 59, 414 (1970).
109. N. J. Turner and R. D. Battershell, Contrib. Boyce Thompson Inst. 24, 139 (1969).
110. C. G. Swain and E. C. Lupton, Jr., J. Amer. Chem. Soc. 90, 4328 (1968).
111. R. L. Jones, R. L. Metcalf, and T. R. Fukuto, J. Econ. Entomol. 62, 801 (1969).
112. T. R. Fukuto, R. L. Metcalf, R. L. Jones, and R. O. Myers, J. Agr. Food Chem. 17, 923 (1969).
113. N. Kakeya, M. Aoki, A. Kamada, and N. Yata, Chem. Pharm. Bull. (Tokyo) 17, 1010 (1969).
114. Y. C. Martin, J. Med. Chem. 13, 145 (1970).
115. A. Wohl, Mol. Pharmacol. 6, 189 (1970).
116. A. Wohl, Mol. Pharmacol. 6, 195 (1970).
117. W. B. Neely, H. C. White, and A. Rudzik, J. Pharm. Sci. 57, 1176 (1968).
118. A. Cammarata, J. Med. Chem, 12, 314 (1969).
119. A. Cammarata, in Molecular Orbital Studies in Chemical Pharmacology, L. B. Kier, Ed., p. 156, Springer-Verlag, New York, 1970.
120. K. S. Rogers and A. Cammarata, Biochim. Biophys. Acta 193, 22 (1969).
121. K. S. Rogers and A. Cammarata, J. Med. Chem. 12, 692 (1969).
122. A. Cammarata, J. Med. Chem. 11, 1111 (1968).
123. A. Cammarata and R. L. Stein, J. Med. Chem. 11, 829 (1968).
124. R. B. Hermann, H. W. Culp, R. E. McMahon, and M. M. Marsh, J. Med. Chem. 12, 749 (1969).
125. G. E. Bass, D. R. Hudson, J. E. Parker, and W. P. Purcell, J. Med. Chem. 14, in press.
126. R. L. O'Brien and F. E. Hahn, Antimicrobial Agents and Chemotherapy-1965, 315 (1966).
127. J. A. Singer and W. P. Purcell, J. Med. Chem. 10, 1000 (1967).
128. V. Nagy and K. Nador, Arnzeim.-Forsch. 17, 1228 (1967).

129. M. Cocordano, C. R. Acad. Sci. Paris, Ser. C. 266, 897 (1968).
130. M. A. Mainster and J. D. Memory, Biochim. Biophys. Acta 148, 605 (1967).
131. W. P. Purcell and K. Sundaram, J. Med. Chem. 12, 18 (1969).
132. N. E. Sharpless and C. L. Greenblatt, Exp. Parasitol. 24, 216 (1969).
133. P. R. Andrews, J. Med. Chem. 12, 761 (1969).
134. W. Perkow, Arzneim.-Forsch. 10, 284 (1960).
135. O. Jardetzky, Adv. Chem. Phys. 7, 499 (1964).
136. O. Jardetzky, Naturwissenschaften 54, 149 (1967).
137. G. Kato, Mol. Pharmacol. 5, 148 (1969).
138. P. G. Schmidt, G. R. Stark, and J. D. Baldeschwiele J. Biol. Chem. 244, 1860 (1969).
139. D. P. Hollis, Biochemistry 6, 2080 (1967).
140. M. A. Raftery, F. W. Dahlquist, S. M. Parsons, and R. G. Wolcott, Proc. Nat. Acad. Sci. U. S. 62, 44 (1969).
141. J. J. Fischer and M. C. Jost, Mol. Pharmacol. 5, 420 (1969).
142. A. Burger, in Fundamental Concepts in Drug-Receptor Interactions, J. F. Danielli, J. F. Moran, and D. J Triggle, Eds., p. 1, Academic Press, New York, 1970
143. E. Schrödinger, Ann. Physik 70, 361 (1926).

CHAPTER II

LINEAR FREE ENERGY-RELATED MODELS: THEORY AND DESCRIPTION

THE FATE OF A DRUG

In living systems, a drug is administered by introducing it, by any one of a number of means, into the natural flow of material which sustains the system. The drug must find its target and destroy, alter, or affect it in some desirable way. One problem that must be faced is that living systems, chemically speaking, present highly reactive environments. First, the amount of administered drug which actually reaches the target might be greatly diminished by such factors as metabolism, localization in other tissues, and removal from the system along with normal waste products. Second, a drug that will kill invading cells or inhibit abnormal processes will also have some effect on normal cells and processes. The true effectiveness of a drug is a measure of its ability to hit the target selectively while leading to only small, acceptable damage to the host. The mode of action, at the molecular level, whereby the drug interacts with the target is seldom well defined and, quite often, is virtually unknown. The reaction of a drug with a target will serve as the basis for the discussion of the theory of the LFER model.

REACTION OF DRUG WITH TARGET SUBSTRATE

Consider the interaction of a drug D with the target biological substrate S:

$$D + S \underset{}{\overset{K}{\rightleftharpoons}} D{:}S \overset{k}{\dashrightarrow} P \qquad \text{(2.1}$$

The drug may be assumed to interact with the substrate to form the complex D:S (more specifically, the "reactive intermediate") which either dissociates back to D and S or goes on to form product P.

The rate of formation of P can be expressed as

$$\frac{d[P]}{dt} = k[D{:}S] \qquad \text{(2.2}$$

Assuming steady-state conditions, one has

$$K = \frac{[D{:}S]}{[D][S]} = \exp(-\Delta G/RT) \qquad \text{(2.3}$$

where ΔG is the Gibbs free energy of formation of the com plex. Solving for [D:S] and substituting into Equation 2.2 gives

$$\frac{d[P]}{dt} = k[D][S][\exp(-\Delta G/RT)] \qquad \text{(2.4}$$

When this expression is integrated from zero product and time to some specified values [P*] and t*, one obtains

$$P^* = k[D][S][\exp(-\Delta G/RT)]\ t^* \qquad \text{(2.5}$$

At this point it should be recognized that [D] represents the drug concentration at the active site and, thus, in practice, is an unknown quantity. To circumvent this problem it is commonly assumed that [D] is proportional to the concentration of the drug administered $[\underline{D}]$, i.e., $[D] = A[\underline{D}]$ where A is less than unity. Employing this approximation leads to

$$P^* = k\ A\ [\underline{D}^*][S][\exp(-\Delta G/RT)]\ t^* \qquad \text{(2.6}$$

where $[\underline{D}^*]$ is the dosage which must be administered in order to produce product [P*] in time t*. If Equation 2.6 is solved for $1/[\underline{D}^*]$ and the base 10 logarithm is taken of each side one obtains

$$\log 1/[\underline{D}^*] = \log A + \log [S] - 0.4343\frac{\Delta G}{RT} + \log \tau^*/P^* \qquad \text{(2.7}$$

The quantity $[\underline{D}^*]$ is a very familiar measure of effective ness; it is often expressed as "LD_{50}," "ID_{25}," "Minimum

Effective Therapeutic Dose," etc. (1). In Equation 2.7, this experimentally determined quantity is expressed as a function of (a) the ability of the drug to reach the target substrate, (b) the target substrate concentration, (c) the ability of the drug to complex with the target, and (d) the rate at which this complex leads to products. Here "products" may broadly be taken to be inhibition of the normal functioning of S, death of the organism, and so on.

This expression (2.7) is of little use if one is interested in the activity of a single drug only. It simply is not practical (and probably not even feasible) to determine experimentally the quantities A, [S], ΔG, and k. One can be satisfied, however, by something less than the prediction from such basic parameters, of the absolute biological activity of some particular compound. Indeed, it would be a significant accomplishment to predict the relative activity of an untested drug which is an analog of an entire series. In this situation, Equation 2.7 can be used to advantage.

Suppose one has a series of n drugs D_1, D_2, . . .D_n which are all similar in chemical structure and all elicit a particular biological response (BR_1, BR_2 . . .BR_n) via the same mechanism. Under these conditions, the quantities k, [S], and (t*/P*) do not vary on going from one drug to the next. Thus, one is able to write

$$\log 1/[\underline{D}(I)] = \log A(I) - \frac{\Delta G(I)}{RT} + C \quad I = 1,n \qquad (2.8)$$

where $[\underline{D}(I)]$ is the administered concentration of drug D_I with corresponding quantities A(I) and $\Delta G(I)$ and C is a constant. These represent a series of n linear equations. In order for them to be useful, the quantities A(I) and $\Delta G(I)$ must be reexpressed in terms of physicochemical properties of the drugs which can be measured or calculated.

In this treatment, the pre-exponential factor A has been introduced as a measure of the ability of a particular drug to move from the point of introduction into the biosystem to the location of the substrate target. In complex living systems, one must assume that in its search for the target, the drug molecule will be required to cross any number of phase boundaries (e.g., membranes), be adsorbed and desorbed from various macromolecules, and, to some extent, eliminated from the system (by excretion or metabolism), or localized in some particular nonreactive region.

As a measure of the potential of a given drug to overcome these obstacles, Hansch and co-workers (2) have introduced and extensively used the approximation

$$A = \exp\left[-\alpha(\pi-\pi°)^2/\beta\right] \qquad (2.9)$$

where π represents the base 10 logarithm of the octanol-water partition coefficient and α and β are constants.

Although the genesis of this expression was originally intuitive and empirical, theoretical treatments based on the probability of a molecule of given partition coefficient transversing alternating aqueous and lipophylic phases has tended to affirm the appropriateness of the early assumptions (3). It should be pointed out that other measures of transportability [e.g., π measured in other solvent systems (4), R_m values from thin-layer chromatography (5), i.e., (6)] should suffice equally well. At this time, perhaps the best reasons for selecting the octanol-water partition coefficients are the relative ease of experimental determination for a very wide variety of classes of compounds and the presence of very large, mutually consistent collections of these data in the literature today. Further, one can quite often calculate approximate π values by assuming substituent additivity, i.e., $\pi = \Sigma_j \pi_j$ where the π_j are atom or group substituent constants derived from measured partition coefficients. This latter procedure is not without pitfalls, however. The most pronounced failures of additivity seem to occur for molecules capable of intramolecular hydrogen bonding (7). In addition to general transport, log P is also interpreted as a measure of the ability of the molecule (or, using π, a particular segment of the molecule) to participate in hydrophobic bonding (8). Accordingly, a quadratic dependence on log P (or π) is usually interpreted as indicating the importance of transport while a linear dependence is taken to imply an important role for hydrophobic bonding in the manifestation of biological activity. It has been pointed out, however, that hydrophobic interactions should be based on ΔH and ΔS and not simply on ΔG (9,10). Further, octanol-water partitioning reflects more than simple hydrophobic bonding, i.e., hydrogen bonding and van der Waals interactions (11,12).

The ΔG term reflects the ability of a given drug to form the requisite activated complex with the target biological substrate. A number of factors can conceivably come into play here. In particular, the activated complex may involve hydrophobic bonding, electrostatic bonding, charge transfer complex formation, or the potential to undergo nucleophilic, electrophilic or redox reactions, and so on.

Since the drug partition coefficient is a measure of the tendency of the drug to move from an aqueous to a non-aqueous phase, it is only natural that π has evolved as a measure of the importance of hydrophobic bonding. A particularly good example of this was reported by Hansch et al. for the binding of phenols to BSA (8). It must be borne in mind constantly, however, that π also quite often parallels other molecular properties, such as size and molecular weight. Again, other parameters, such as R_m, should also be of use. Indeed, Rogers and Cammarata (13) have demonstrated that, for some classes of agents, certain quantum mechanical indices can be closely correlated with π.

Electrostatic interaction between molecules can be treated at several different levels of sophistication. In general, each molecule may be considered to be a collection of relatively fixed charges. The interaction energy will contain charge-charge, charge-dipole, dipole-dipole, etc. contributions as well as London dispersion forces (14). Thus, theoretically calculated charge distributions (15,16) and experimental dipole moments (17) have been used as measures of the ability of a drug to form an electrostatic complex.

The Hammett equation (18,19) provides a time-honored free energy-related relationship between reaction rates (particularly ester hydrolysis) and the electronic effect of substituents. In particular,

$$\log (k_o) = \rho\sigma \qquad (2.10)$$

where k_o is the rate (or equilibrium) constant for parent compound (i.e., a benzoic acid ester) and k is the corresponding constant for a derivation involving (most properly) meta or para substitutions on the phenyl ring. The ionization of benzoic acid has been chosen as a standard reaction for which ρ is fixed at 1.00. A positive σ value for a particular substituent indicates that the substituent is a stronger electron attractor than hydrogen, while a negative σ value implies a weaker electron attractor than hydrogen. Reactions with positive ρ values are aided by electron withdrawal from the benzene ring, whereas those with negative ρ values are made more difficult by electron withdrawal.

Reaction types which have been studied include ionization of benzoic acids, phenols, and amines; hydrolysis of alkyl benzoates and benzyl chlorides; benzoylation of aromatic amines; reduction of nitro benzenes; addition of HCN to benzaldehydes; side chain bromination of acetophenones; and decomposition of substituted benzoyl peroxides (19,20).

The rationale for the Hammett relationship lies in that log K_{eq} for a reaction is proportional to the standard free-energy change, $\Delta G°$, and that log k_{rate} is proportional, in the framework of the transition-state theory, to the free energy of activation. Using the approach introduced by Taft (21,22), this type of work has been extended to study aliphatic compounds as well (23).

Electronic indices from molecular orbital calculations may serve to point out the relative abilities of a series of drug analogs to undergo a particular reaction (24-26). The electron charge distribution has been used (with and without success) as a measure of the susceptibility of the atoms in the molecule to chemical attack. Electrophilic attack should occur at the point of largest negative charge density, while nucleophilic attack should occur at the point of largest positive charge for the molecule in its ground state.

The "frontier electron theory" is somewhat related to the charge density. The ability of a molecule to undergo nucleophilic attack is postulated to be related to the ability of the unoccupied orbitals of the molecule to accommodate the approaching electron pair of the attacking agent. The likelihood of attack occurring at some particular atom Y in the molecule is related to the capacity of the unoccupied orbital in the region of that atom. Two parameters, the frontier electron density (f_Y^N) and the super delocalizability (S_Y^N), are defined in equations 2.11 and 2.12:

$$f_Y^N = 2C_i(Y)^2 \qquad (2.11)$$

$$S_Y^N = 2\sum_{j=i}^{m} C_j(Y)^2/E_j \qquad (2.12)$$

Here i identifies the lowest empty molecular orbital, $C_i(Y)$ is the coefficient of the *i*th MO at the atom Y, E_j is the energy of the *j*th MO, and the summation runs from i = lowest empty MO to m the highest empty MO. Corresponding quantities can be defined for electrophilic and radical attack.

It is conceivable that any one or several of a number of parameters might be used to establish the relative

ΔG values governing the critical (rate determining) steps in some given biological response. Thus, one might consider the general expression analogous to Equation 2.8:

$$\log (1/D_i^*) = a_1P_1(i) + a_2P_2(i) + a_3P_3(i) + \ldots + a_mP_m(i) + C \quad (2.13)$$

Here $P_1(i) \ldots P_m(i)$ represent m different, linearly independent physicochemical parameters required to characterize the dependence of the activity of the *i*th drug on A_i and ΔG_i. If for each analog in a series of n drugs one has experimental or calculated values for each of the parameters $P_1 \ldots P_m$ where m<n, then numerical values for the constants $a_1, a_2, \ldots a_m$ and C can be obtained by multiple regression analysis. One obtains the set of values for which the sum of the squares of the deviations of log $(1/\underline{D}_i^*)$ calculated using Equation 2.13 from the corresponding experimentally derived quantities is a minimum.

Equation 2.13 is perfectly general. The Hansch expression, namely,

$$\log (1/C) = a\pi^2 + b\pi + \rho\sigma + cE_s + d \quad (2.14)$$

may be considered to be specific example of 2.13 in which one considers transport, π, electronic, σ, and steric, E_s (27), properties.

The result of such an analysis can be used in two ways. If for some untested analog one obtains values for the $P_1 \ldots P_m$, one can calculate a predicted biological activity. Also, correlation of activity within a closely similar series of molecules with specific physicochemical parameters often sheds some light on the mode of action. For a good review on this subject, the reader is referred to the works by McFarland (28).

STATISTICAL CONSIDERATIONS

The extent to which one is able to answer questions of either type depends on the "goodness of fit" of the theoretical model to the data. If one seeks to correlate the biological activities of n compounds with a total of m physicochemical properties of these compounds, statistical measures of goodness of fit can be employed as long as $n > m + 1$. Naturally, the larger the excess of experimental BR's over the number of physicochemical parameters, the better one is able to determine the goodness of fit. There are a number of statistics which may be used in conjunction with quantitative structure-activity analysis; each focuses on a slightly different aspect of the goodness of fit. For this reason, several statistics are usually applied (16,29,30).

For notational simplicity, let the regression equations (2.13) be rewritten as

$$\hat{Y}_i = \sum_{j=1}^{m} A_j X_{ij} + C \qquad i = 1,2 \ldots n \tag{2.15}$$

where $\hat{Y}_i$ is an estimate of the experimentally determined quantity Y_i which is the observed biological response of the *i*th compound in the series of n analogs, X_{ij} is the value of the *j*th particular parameter (such as the Hammett σ value) for that compound, A_j is the coefficient for the *j*th parameter, c is a constant, and m is the total number of physicochemical parameters included in the analysis.

The values of the a_j, j = 1,m, and c are determined so that they minimize the sum of the squares of the deviations of Y_i (the actual experimentally determined values) from $\hat{Y}_i$ (the calculated values) i.e., $\sum_{i=1}^{n} (Y_i - \hat{Y}_i)^2$. These coefficients can be shown to be unbiased and have the smallest standard errors of any such set that are linear expressions of the Y's. The standard deviation for the equation is given as

$$[\sum_{i=1} (Y_i - \hat{Y}_i)^2/(n-1)]^{1/2} \tag{2.16}$$

An often-used statistic is the "multiple correlation coefficient," R (31). This measure of goodness of fit is useful when one desires to examine the joint relation of Y with the X variables, taken all together. It is defined as the simple correlation coefficient between Y and its linear regression. Since it would be difficult to attach a useful meaning to the sign of R, most applications deal with its square, expressed as

$$R^2 = \sum_{i=1}^{n} (\hat{Y}_i - \bar{Y})^2 / \sum_{i=1}^{n} (Y_i - \bar{Y})^2 \tag{2.17}$$

where

$$\bar{Y} = \sum_{i=1}^{n} Y_i/n$$

i.e., the average value of the Y's. Accordingly, R^2 is the fraction of the sum of squares of deviations of Y from its mean that is attributable to the regression. One might note that, in the event of perfect fit, i.e., $Y_i = \hat{Y}_i$ for all i, R^2 will take on its maximum value, unity. The poorer the fit, the closer R^2 will approach its minimum value, zero. R^2 is one of the most commonly reported statistics in QSAR studies.

One may approach the question of goodness of fit by asking if there does indeed exist a linear relationship between Y_i and the X_{ij} such that all of the coefficients, A_j, are significantly different from zero. Such a test of the null hypothesis that the multiple correlation in the population is zero is provided by the F-test, sometimes referred to as the F-ratio or F (overall). This statistic is defined by

$$F = (n - k - 1)R^2/k(1-R^2) \qquad (2.18)$$

where $F = [\Sigma(\hat{Y}_i - \bar{Y}_i)^2/(k - 1)]/\Sigma(Y_i - \hat{Y}_i)^2/(n - k)]$ with (k - 1) and (n - k) degrees of freedom, where k = m + 1 (32). The value calculated for F can be used to obtain the corresponding significance level from a table of F distributions (33). For example, given n = 20 and k = 3, F = 7.26 would correspond to a probability of less than 1% that the null hypothesis is valid (all coefficients = 0) or, alternatively, that the regression is significant at the 99% level.

In QSAR studies, one is often as interested in understanding the variation in biological response from one compound to the next as one is in obtaining simply an empirical expression from which biological responses for additional compounds can be calculated. For example, for a particular problem one might wish to know if the observed activity variations can best be associated with a transport parameter (such as Hansch's π), an electronic parameter (such as the Hammett σ), or a combination of the two. The multiple correlation coefficient is not very helpful in making such a decision. It is always true that the more parameters one includes in the regression analysis, the higher (more favorable) the value calculated for R^2 will be. Inspection of the formula for R^2 will reveal that no dependence on the degrees of freedom appears therein.

A statistic which may be described as the "explained variance," EV, is very useful in such situations (34). EV is obtained by subtracting the ratio of the deviations mean square, $\Sigma_{i=1}^{N} (\hat{Y}_i - Y_i)^2/(n-k)$, to the mean square of Y, $\Sigma_{i=1}^{N} (Y_i - \bar{Y}_i)^2/(n-1)$, from unity, i.e.,

$$EV = 1 - \frac{\Sigma (\hat{Y}_i - Y_i)^2/(n-k)}{\Sigma (Y_i - \bar{Y}_i)^2/(n-1)} \quad (2.19)$$

This quantity is an estimate of the fraction of the variance that is "explained" by the X variables and reflects the number of degrees of freedom in the analysis. It is not uncommon to find a decrease in EV on going from an equation containing m parameters to one containing m + 1. One should note that in the event of perfect fit, $\hat{Y}_i = Y_i$ for all i, the maximum value for EV, unity, will be obtained. Unlike R^2, however, negative values for EV are possible. This will occur when the average Y value, $\bar{Y}$, provides, on a per-degree-of-freedom basis, a better approximation to the observed values, Y_i, than do the calculated values, $\hat{Y}_i$.

The significance of the individual coefficients, A_j, can be established using Students' t-test (35). The null hypothesis that the jth coefficient, A_j, is zero can be tested by computing t_j, the ratio of A_j to its standard error, S_{A_j}. Confidence limits for the coefficients, at, for example, the 95% level are found as $A_j \pm t_{0.05}S_{A_j}$ where $t_{0.05}$ is the tabulated t value corresponding to the 95% confidence level with n - 1 degrees of freedom. Alternatively, the value for t_j with n - 1 degrees of freedom can be used to obtain the corresponding significance level for that coefficient from a table of critical values of Students' t-distribution (36).

For additional reading in the area of statistics, including the concept of variance, the reader is referred to the books by Moroney (37) and Hinchen (38).

Of great importance as a precaution to the statistical interpretation of the results of QSAR studies by multiple regression analysis is the recent work of Topliss and Costello (39). Although the number of degrees of freedom in any statistical correlation is obviously important, a point which is sometimes overlooked is the influence of the total number of independent variables screened for possible correlation with activity on the statistical significance of the resulting correlation. The greater the number of variables tested, the greater the role chance will play in the observed correlation.

By using random numbers, Topliss and Costello studied the degree of chance correlation in such QSAR studies as a function of the number of observations, the overall number of variables tested, and the number of these variables actually included in each analysis. The results of their study are given in Figures 2.1 and 2.2.

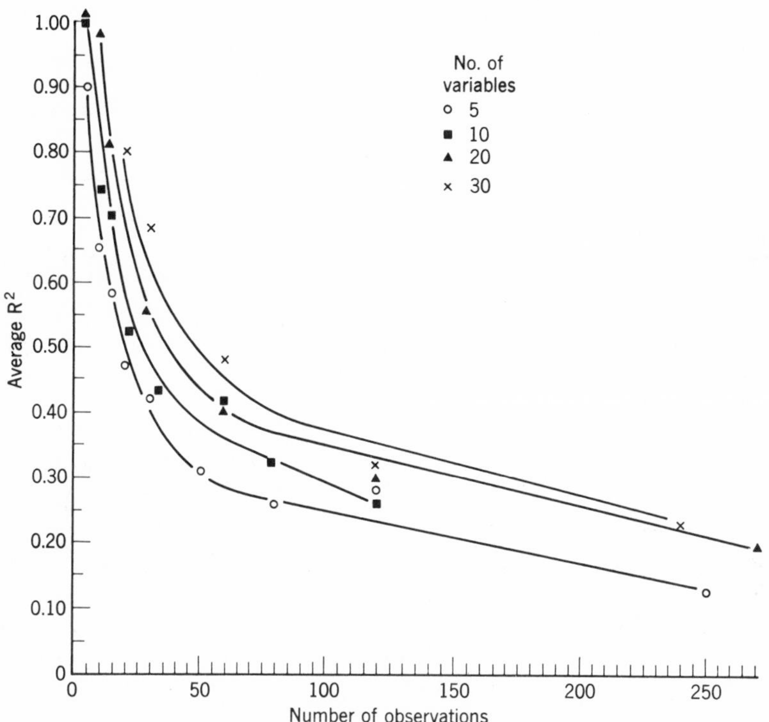

Figure 2.1. Relationship between R^2 and number of observations.

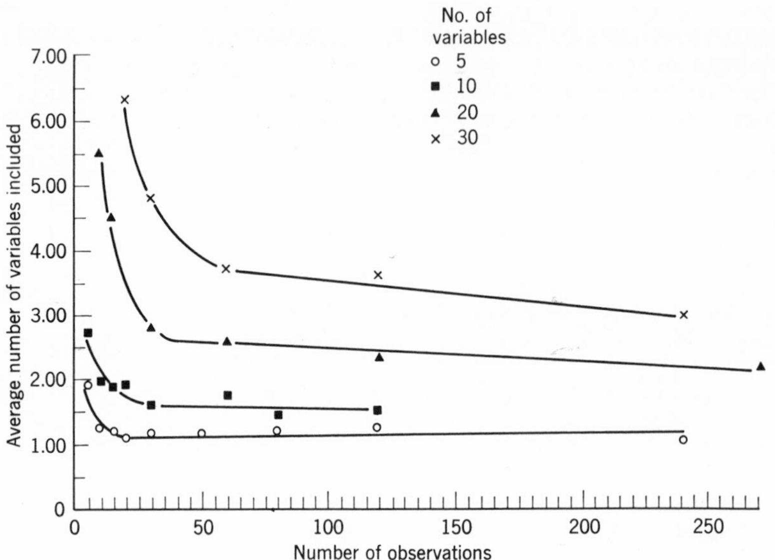

Figure 2.2. Relationship between mean number of variable and number of observations.

In Figure 2.1 the average r^2 values from 100 trials are plotted against the number of observations (dependent variables) for various fixed numbers of independent variables tested. From this plot, it is apparent that impres sive chance correlations were obtained when the number of observations was small relative to the number of independent variables tested. All variables were significant at a minimum of the 90% confidence level. With an increasin number of observations, the degree of chance correlation was steadily reduced.

The relationship between the mean number of independent variables included in an equation and the number of observations for different fixed numbers of variables tested is illustrated in Figure 2.2. It shows that the number of variables correlating by chance increases as the number of observations decreases.

Also, for a given number of observations, the number of variables included in a particular equation must increase as the number of variables tested increases.

This study affirms a potential problem of considerable magnitude in QSAR correlations where many possible variables must be considered. This problem may be particularly important in MO-type correlations where many different parameters may be calculated for a particular compound and where there is no apparent reason to choose one parameter over another. In the Free-Wilson procedure this phenomenon does not arise since the statistical analysis takes a different form. Thus, it is extremely important to be aware of the ratio of independent variables to dependent variables in view of the problem of chance correlations. To reduce adequately the risk of chance, a large number of observations are needed. However, these are not always available. Certainly those correlations are essentially meaningless in which the number of possible variables approach or equal the number of observations.

Topliss and Costello estimate that if $r^2 = 0.40$ is regarded as the maximum acceptable level of chance correlation, then the minimum number of observations required to test five independent variables is about 30, for 10 variables 40 observations, for 20 variables 65 observations, and for 30 variables 80 observations.

INTERPRETATIONS

As is true in all model systems, the real value of the LFER lies in its ability to be applied to a particular problem of interest. Due to the wide variety of parameters that may be used in such an analysis, the potential of the method is great in the elucidation of the mechanism of drug action and in drug design per se. For example, the analysis may demonstrate the importance of hydrophobic forces and clarify the nature of these hydrophobic interactions in eliciting a particular response from a selected drug. Statistical significance of the π^2, π, or other hydrophobic parameters might indicate its important influence in affecting the random walk of the drug to its site of action, the orientation of the drug on an enzyme or receptor, and the possible allosteric transition of the enzyme or receptor. On the other hand, application of steric factors to structure-activity analyses may also aid in the elucidation of the mechanism of drug action. Although most steric parameters are used to approximate intramolecular, and not intermolecular, steric interactions, the study of increasingly larger substituents may find a point at which the substituent effect relationship fails and thus may aid in mapping the free space about an active site. It is also possible that a conformational change effected by a specific substituent is indicated by the failure of that substituent to conform to the equation describing the rest of the series.

Similarly, statistical significance of the electronic term may indicate if there are electronic influences in the mechanism of action of the drugs studied. In addition, the sign of the coefficient associated with that term can indicate whether the receptor site is electrophilic or nucleophilic in nature. For example, the negative coefficient of the electronic term in the study of enzyme inhibitors might suggest that the inhibitors are bound to an electron-deficient site on the enzyme. The particular type of σ constant, if this is used as the electronic parameter, might indicate the molecular position dominant in the drug's electronic interactions. Of course, the correlation obtained with the particular electronic parameter cannot always suggest unambiguously the exact mechanism by which electronic factors operate. Such correlations may aid, however, in the delineation of the relative importance of such parameters in elicitin biological response.

As is true with the Free-Wilson method (Chapter V), the LFER model holds much promise in its application to drug design. Of course, no structure-activity analysis can do more than suggest molecules for synthesis and study. It is conceded that the only way to determine a molecule's activity is through experiment. The application of such an analysis to one series of compounds might suggest the desirability of considering a completely new series of compounds. For example, the negative coefficient of the hydrophobic term in the analysis of one series of drugs might indicate that the parent side chain are too lipophilic for maximum activity. This would suggest the consideration of other more hydrophilic (negativ π values) substituent groups.

The LFER analysis might also save needless synthesis and biological evaluation of other compounds by suggestin that the attempt to find a derivative more active than th parent molecule is unlikely to succeed. That is, the analysis of one series of compounds might suggest that th properties most likely to elicit a maximum pharmacological response are already contained within that series. A third application of the Hansch analysis in drug design is its potential to give a new direction to the study by selecting molecules or properties to yield more potent compounds. For example, the first derivative of Equation 2.14 with respect to π yields the maximum or ideal value of π, π_o (40). The use of π_o or log P_o may suggest a starting point for the design of a new series of drugs for a specific action if the hydrophobic term is statistically significant for biological activity.

Examples of successful predictions of activity are becoming less rare, but one of the first successes using a LFER model was reported by Fuller, Marsh, and Mills (41). They predicted the inhibitory potency of two N-(phenoxyethyl)cyclopropylamine derivatives against monoamine oxidase.

REFERENCES

1. G. A. Condouris, Drill's Pharmacology in Medicine, 3rd ed., J. R. DiPalmo, Ed., McGraw-Hill Book Co., New York, 1965, Chapter 2.
2. C. Hansch and T. Fujita, J. Amer. Chem. Soc. 86, 1616 (1963).
3. C. Hansch, Acc. Chem. Res. 2, 232 (1969).
4. T. Fujita, J. Iwasa, and C. Hansch, J. Amer. Chem. Soc. 86, 5175 (1964).
5. G. L. Biagi, M. C. Guerra, A. M. Barbaro, and M. F. Gamba, J. Med. Chem. 13, 511 (1970).
6. A. Leo, C. Hansch, and C. Church, J. Med. Chem. 12, 766 (1969).
7. C. Hansch and S. M. Anderson, J. Org. Chem. 32, 2583 (1967).
8. C. Hansch, K. Kiehs, and G. L. Lawrence, J. Amer. Chem. Soc. 87, 5770 (1965).
9. A. Canas-Rodriguez and M. S. Tute, 161st National Meeting, Amer. Chem. Soc., March 1971, Abstracts of Papers, PEST 51.
10. W. Kauzmann, Advan. Protein Chem. 14, 37 (1959).
11. S. Rajender and R. Lumry, 161st National Meeting, Amer. Chem. Soc., March 1971, Abstracts of Papers, PEST 52.
12. C. Hansch, J. E. Quinlan, and G. L. Lawrence, J. Org. Chem. 33, 347 (1968).
13. K. E. Rogers and A. Cammarata, J. Med. Chem. 12, 692 (1969).
14. J. O. Hirschfelder, Molecular Biophysics, Weissbluth and Pullman, Eds., p. 325, Academic Press Inc., New York, 1965.
15. W. P. Purcell, J. Med. Chem, 9, 294 (1966).
16. G. E. Bass, D. R. Hudson, J. E. Parker, and W. P. Purcell, J. Med. Chem. 14, 275 (1971).
17. W. P. Purcell, J. G. Beasley, and R. P. Quintana, Biochim. Biophys. Acta 88, 233 (1964).
18. L. P. Hammett, J. Amer. Chem. Soc. 59, 96 (1937).
19. L. P. Hammett, Trans. Faraday Soc. 34, 156 (1938).
20. H. H. Jaffé, Chem. Rev. 53, 191 (1953).
21. R. W. Taft, Jr., J. Amer. Chem. Soc. 74, 2729 (1952)
22. R. W. Taft, Jr., J. Amer. Chem. Soc. 74, 3120 (1952)
23. J. E. Leffler and E. Grunwald, Rates and Equilibria Of Organic Reactions, John Wiley and Sons, Inc., New York, 1963.
24. A. Pullman and B. Pullman, Quantum Biochemistry, Interscience Publishers, 1963.

25. A. Streitweiser, Molecular Orbital Theory for the Organic Chemist, John Wiley and Sons, Inc., New York, 1961.
26. L. Salem, Molecular Orbital Theory of Conjugated Systems, W. A. Benjamin, Inc., New York, 1966.
27. C. Hansch, A. R. Steward, S. M. Anderson, and D. Bentley, J. Med. Chem. 11, 1 (1968).
28. J. W. McFarland, in Progress in Drug Research, E. Tucker, Ed., Vol. 15, p. 123, Birkhäuser Verlag, Basel, 1971.
29. P. N. Craig, C. H. Hansch, J. W. McFarland, Y. C. Martin, W. P. Purcell, and R. Zahradnik, J. Med. Chem. 14, 447 (1971).
30. G. W. Snedecor and W. G. Cochran, Statistical Methods, 6th ed., Chap. 13, p. 381, The Iowa State Univ. Press, Ames, Iowa, 1967.
31. Ibid. p. 402.
32. Ibid. pp. 385-387.
33. Ibid. pp. 560-567.
34. Ibid. p. 386.
35. Ibid. p. 138.
36. Ibid. p. 549.
37. M. J. Moroney, Facts from Figures, Penguin Books, Baltimore, Md., 1951.
38. J. D. Hinchen, Practical Statistics for Chemical Research, Methuen and Co., Ltd., London, 1969.
39. J. G. Topliss and R. J. Costello, J. Med. Chem, in press.
40. C. Hansch and T. Fujita, J. Amer. Chem. Soc. 86, 1616 (1964).
41. R. W. Fuller, M. M. Marsh, and J. Mills. J. Med. Chem. 11, 397 (1968).

CHAPTER III

LINEAR FREE ENERGY-RELATED MODELS: APPLICATIONS AND PARAMETERS

The more physicochemically useful model of the two QSAR methods is the LFER model of Hansch. As outlined in Chapter II, this more widely used method attributes the biological response of a given drug to some combination of its hydrophobic, electronic, and steric properties. By approximating these physicochemical properties with measured or theoretical values, one may be able to use the method as an aid to determine the relativ importance and role of each factor in the biological mech anism. This is usually approached by studying a series of closely related molecules and a given biological activity.

Unlike the few reported examples of the Free-Wilson mathematical model, literature applications of the Hansch method are numerous. Since the initial introduction of the model in 1963, illustrations of the applications and modifications of it have mushroomed to the point that they appear frequently in the literature (1-10). Not surprisingly, Hansch and co-workers have easily dominated the literature with their examples of the method. Following their initial proposal of the technique (11,12), this group has applied the basic ρ-σ-π equation (3.1) or modifications of it (3.2-3.5) to all sorts of drugs and biological systems (2.4, 5, 11-41):

$$\log (1/C) = -a\pi^2 + b\pi + \rho\sigma + c \qquad (3.1)$$

$$\log (1/C) = -a\pi^2 + b\pi + c \qquad (3.2)$$

$$\log (1/C) = b\pi + c \quad (3.3)$$

$$\log (1/C) = b\pi + \rho\sigma + c \quad (3.4)$$

$$\log (1/C) = \rho\sigma + c$$

In Equations 3.1-3.5, C is the molar concentration of the compound necessary to elicit a defined level of biological response; π is the hydrophobic substituent parameter (including some steric factors) defined as the difference between the logarithm of the partition coefficient of the parent unsubstituted compound and that of its derivative (for the experimental details of partition coefficient measurement recommended by Hansch, the reader is referred to Appendix I); σ is the Hammett substituent parameter which is a measure of the electronic effect on reaction rate; and a, b, c, and ρ are constants generated by the regression analysis. Most of these examples have yielded statistically significant correlations between the physicochemical parameters of the molecules and their elicited responses.

In addition to the original π-σ parameter approximations of hydrophobic, steric, and electronic factors involved in drug action, the use of many other such parameters has been suggested. In 1963 Hansch and co-workers initiated the use of the logarithms of the partition coefficients (P) of the entire molecules to approximate hydrophobic, and to a limited degree steric, factors in place of the substituent π parameter (12); numerous applications of this parameter have since been made (Table 3.1). They have also suggested the use of the chromatographic parameter R_M (37,42) and McGowan's parachor [P] or adjusted parachor [P*] rather than π in such studies since they have been shown to be additive as well as related to π. R_M is defined as $(1-R_F)/R_F$ where R_F is the quotient of the distance moved by the compound divided by that moved by the solvent on a chromatogram. The substituent chromatographic constant, ΔR_f (R_M of the substituted compound $-R_M$ of the unsubstituted compound), has also been successfully used (4,37). Another estimate of the hydrophobic factors involved in eliciting pharmacological responses which has been used in QSAR studies is the solubility parameter, δ, and its logarithm, log δ. The logarithms of the water and chloroform solubilities, log S_W and log S_C, respectively, have also been utilized in LFER studies.

Table 3.1 summarizes some parameters which have been used in the Hansch analysis.

Table 3.1 Hydrophobic Parameters Used in the Linear Free Energy-Related Model

Symbol	Parameter	Reference
π, π^2	Hansch-Fujita substituent hydrophobic constant	2-5, 11-17 19-22, 24, 26-41, 48, 50-79
log P, (log P)^2	Logarithm of partition coefficient	3-5, 11, 12 20, 21, 23, 24, 26, 32, 33, 36, 37, 40, 53, 68, 69, 75, 80-100
R_M	Chromatographic parameter	42, 88, 101-109
ΔR_M	Substituent chromatographic parameter	4, 37
δ, log δ	Solubility parameter	79, 110-112
log S_w	Logarithm of water solubility	79
log S_c	Logarithm of chloroform solubility	79
[P]	Parachor	113-117
[P*]	Adjusted parachor	113, 118

In attempts to delineate the factors involved in drug-receptor interactions, Hansch has suggested the incorporation of Taft-type steric parameters into the LFER equations (43).

Although there is still some interrelationship between the hydrophobic and steric factors, this does allow isolation of the effects to some degree. The first steri parameter suggested was the Taft substituent steric parameter E_s and successful applications of this parameter have been reported (Table 3.2). More recently, modified

Table 3.2 Steric Parameters Used in Linear Free Energy Related Model

Symbol	Parameter	Reference
E_s	Taft steric parameter	2-5, 13, 17, 18, 21, 23, 24, 26, 28, 30, 33, 39, 43, 48, 68, 76, 83, 119, 120
$E_s^{o,m}$	Modified Taft steric parameter for ortho and meta substituents	38, 39
E_s^p	Modified Taft steric parameters for para substituents	38, 39
E_s^c	Hancock's corrected steric parameter	3, 5, 19, 27
MV	Molar volume	45
r_v	Van der Waal's radius	38, 39, 46, 47
R	Interatomic distances	48, 49
γ	Arbitrarily defined steric parameter of Hermann et al.	50

Taft steric parameters, $E_s^{o,m}$ and E_s^p, have been used for ortho and meta and para substituents, respectively (38, 39). Hancock's corrected steric parameter, E_s^c, also a modification of the Taft E_s, has been successfully applied in the LFER equations (3,5,19,44). Other investigators have used molar volume, M.V. (45), van der Waal's radius, r_v (38,39,46,47), and interatomic distances, R (48,49), to account for steric effects in QSAR studies. Hermann and co-workers have even defined an arbitrary steric constant, γ, to approximate steric factors in their studies (50). A summary of some of the more commonly used steric parameters is given in Table 3.2.

The third major factor, electronic, incorporated in the "extrathermodynamic" model of QSAR studies has been represented by a most diverse set of parameters. Since the initial use of the Hammett σ constants in such studies experimental and theoretical indices have been used to approximate the electronic aspects of drug-receptor interactions. The most widely used parameters include various modifications of the Hammett σ values to describe better a particular situation. These parameters include σ_o (121), σ_m (4,21,27,48,60,122), and σ_p (4,19,34,65,122), which describe the electronic effects of a substituent substituted at the ortho, meta, and para positions, respectively, on a side chain. The σ^+ value has been used for examples in which an electron-withdrawing group interacts with developing a positive charge in the transition state (17,19, 25,122). Similarly, σ^- parameters have been included in situations where an electron-donating group interacts with an intermediate negative charge (2,5,11,15,18,30,123). Following the procedure of Taft in the separation of σ int the inductive and resonance components, several investigators have used σ_I to account for inductive electronic effects (13,19,24,46,48,54,55,124) and σ_R to describe resonance factors (46,54,55). Another widely used parameter analogous to the Hammett σ value is the Taft polar substituent constant σ^* (Table 3.3-A). While σ is used for aromatic systems, σ^* is applied to aliphatic systems. The radical constant, $\sigma^{\cdot}$, has also been utilized in studies of the relative rates of phenylation (19). Craig has include σ_{sc} to describe the electronic effect directed to a side chain (121). The modified Hammett constants, $\sigma^{\cdot}$, of Yoshioka et al. have also been included in the Hansch analyses.

Another widely used electronic parameter is the pK_A value, the negative logarithm of the ionization constant (Table 3.3-A). In addition to the use of pK_A, its substituent parameter ΔpK_A, has also been utilized (3,15,26, 66,67,84). It is defined as the change in the negative logarithm of the ionization constants of the substituted and unsubstituted compounds. Ionization potentials, I (113,137), molar electronic polarizabilities, P_E (24,34, 46,48,54,55), electronic polarizabilities, α (113,137, 139,140,151), electric dipole moments, μ (56,78,88,91), and group dipole moments, m (56,139,140) have also been employed to describe electronic characteristics of drugs in these analyses. Others have approximated this factor with molar attraction constants, F (112), fractional molar attraction constants, f_p (141), reaction equilibrium constants, log k (73), and spectroscopic chemical shifts, γ and Δppm (66, 67,123). Reaction

Table 3.3 Electronic Parameters Used in Linear Free Energy-Related Model

Symbol	Parameter	Reference
A. Experimental parameters		
σ, σ^2	Hammett constant	2-5, 11-18, 21-26, 28-30, 32, 38-41, 46, 47, 50, 51, 54, 55, 58, 60-68, 76, 77, 82, 83, 92, 123, 125-132
σ^-	Electronic effect of substituent at ortho position to side chain	121
σ_m	Electronic effect of substituent at meta position to side chain	4, 21, 27, 28, 60, 122
σ_p	Electronic effect of substituent at para position to side chain	4, 19, 34, 65, 122
σ_I	Taft aliphatic inductive constant	3, 19, 24, 25, 46-48, 54, 55, 120, 124, 128, 130
σ_R	Taft aliphatic resonance constant	46, 54, 55
σ^*	Taft polar substituent constant	3-5, 21, 24,29, 43, 56, 59, 83, 84, 119, 120, 128, 130
σ'	Yoshioka et al. modified Hammett constant	82, 133
σ^+	Enhanced Hammett constant for electron-withdrawing group	17, 19, 25, 122

Table 3.3 Continued

Symbol	Parameter	Reference
σ^-	Enhanced Hammett constant for electron-donating group	2, 5, 11, 15, 18, 30, 123
σ_{sc}	Electronic effect directed to side chain	121
$\sigma\cdot$	Radical constant for relative rate of phenylation	19
pK_A	Negative logarithm of the ionization constant	4, 15, 27, 31, 33, 40, 79, 82, 85, 92, 123, 124, 134-136
ΔpK_A	Change in the negative logarithm of the ionization constants of substituted and unsubstituted compounds	3, 15, 26, 66, 67, 84
I	Ionization potential	113, 137
P_E	Molar electronic polarizability	24, 34, 46, 48 54, 55, 138
α	Electronic polarizability	113, 137, 139, 140
F	Molar attraction constant	112
f_p	Fractional molar attraction constants	141
log k	Reaction equilibrium constant	73
μ	Electric dipole moment	56, 78, 88, 91
m, m^2	Group dipole moment	56, 139, 140
γ, Δppm	Spectroscopic chemical shift	66, 67, 123
$t_{1/2}$	Reaction parameter	73, 107
Δk	Hydrogen bonding parameter	138

Table 3.3 Continued

Symbol	Parameter	Reference
E_R	Homolytic constant	25, 34, 46, 47, 122, 125, 142
$\mathcal{F}$	Inductive field constant	13, 59, 63, 113, 122, 143
$\mathcal{R}$	Resonance constant	13, 59, 63, 122, 143
β	Association to albumin	67
Q	Copolymerization constant	34, 144
σ_i σ_π	Yukawa-Tsumo parameters for estimation of π electron charge density distributions	76, 131, 145, 146
B. Theoretical Quantum Mechanical Indices		
ε	Atomic charge densities	4, 30, 62, 91
q, Q^T, Q	Atomic net charge, total net charge, and absolute value of net charge	71, 81, 97, 147-149
q^σ, Q^σ	Atomic σ electron net charge	81, 149
q^π, Q^π	Atomic π electron net charge	51, 81, 149
S_r^n	Nucleophilic superdelocalizability	5, 55, 81, 145, 146, 150
S_r^E	Electrophilic superdelocalizability	51, 55, 81, 97, 145, 146, 149, 150
S_r^R	Free radical superdelocalizability	145, 146
f	Frontier electron density	71
F_r	Free valance	145, 146

Table 3.3 Continued

Symbol	Parameter	Reference
E_{LEMO},	Energy of the lowest empty molecular orbital	51, 62, 149
E_{HOMO},	Energy of the highest occupied molecular orbital	92, 149
Δf_r	Valence force constants	66, 67, 123
c	Atomic orbital coefficient	71, 55, 147
δ_c	Occupation number	62
Δ_E	Difference in eigenvalues	62
δ_E	Incipient-transition-state differences	62
Θ	Total interaction energy	50
$\pi'_{N,N}$	Frontier self-atom polarizability	149
$\pi'_{N,N+1}$	Frontier atom-atom polarizability	149
$F^{[A]}$	Intermolecular Coulombic interaction energy	149
$E^{[A]}$	Electric field created at point [A] by a set of charges on a molecule	149

parameters which have been used with some degree of success include the homolytic constants, E_R (25,34,46,47, 122,125,142), hydrogen bonding parameters, Δk (138), inductive field and resonance constants, $\mathcal{F}$ (13,59,63,113, 122,143), and $\mathcal{R}$ (13,59,63,122,143), respectively, association to albumin parameters, β (67), and copolymerization constants, Q (34,144). Sasaki and Suzuki have applied Yukawa and Tsuno's σ_i and σ_π parameters for the approximation of the π electron charge density distribution in an extrathermodynamic analysis. These parameters are summarized in Section A of Table 3.3.

In addition to these "experimental" electronic parameters, the integration of molecular orbital calculations with QSAR analyses has resulted in many "theoretical" electronic constants derived from quantum mechanical indices (Table 3.3-B). Using the results obtained from various levels of approximation of quantum mechanical calculations, investigators have applied atomic charge density values, ε (4,30,62,91), total atomic net charges, q and Q^T (71,81,97,147-149), atomic σ-electron net charge values, q^σ and Q^σ (81,149) and atomic π-electron net charges, q^π and Q^π (51,81,149) to the Hansch-type equations. Nucleophilic, electrophilic, and free radical superdelocalizability indices, S_r^n, S_r^E, and S_r^R, respectively, have also been used to explain electronic drug-receptor interactions (150) (Table 3.3-B). Frontier electron density values, f (71), free valences, F_r (145, 146), valence force constants, Δf_r (66,67,123), and atomic orbital coefficients, c (55,71,147), have also been used successfully. Hermann et al. have studied the use of the value of the energy of the lowest empty molecular orbital, E_{LEMO}, occupation numbers, δc, eigenvalue difference, Δ_E, and incipient-transition-state differences, δ_E, in LFER equations (62). In addition, Fuller has employed the total interaction energy term, Θ, in similar studies (50). Further examples by Wohl included the use of E_{HOMO}, the energy level of the highest occupied molecular orbital; $\pi_{N,N'}$ the frontier self-atom polarizability of atom N; $\pi_{N',N+1'}$ the frontier atom-atom polarizability between atoms N and N + 1; F[A], the intermolecular coulombic interaction energy for a molecule and point [A]; and E[A], the electric field created at point [A] by a set of charges on a molecule, in the Hansch analysis (149). In addition, many of these same indices have been used in attempts to explain the physical interpretation of LFER in biological systems (55) and the quantum chemical relationship to partitioning properties (132,148). Table 3.3-B summarizes the various quantum mechanical indices which have been utilized as electronic parameters in the LFER model.

In addition to the hydrophobic, steric, and electronic parameters, several miscellaneous properties or combinations of other parameters have been used in the Hansch analysis. As summarized in Table 3.4, these include the molecular weight of the compound, M.W. (79,113); an arbitrary group contribution (47); the number of carbon atoms that comprise the substituent, N (138,152); the number of hydrogen atoms attached to a certain atom, n_H (27,92); and the vapor pressure of the compound, V.P.

Table 3.4 Miscellaneous Parameters Used in the Linear Free Energy-Related Model

Symbol	Parameter	Reference
M.W.	Molecular weight	79, 113
	Group Contribution	47
N	Number of carbon atoms in a substituent	138, 152
n_H	Number of hydrogen atoms attached	27, 92
V.P.	Vapor pressure	107
πF	Product of hydrophobic and molar attraction constants	112
ε log P	Product of partitioning and atomic charge density values	33
log Pσ*	Logarithm of product of partitioning and electronic parameters	84
log σ* log P	Product of logarithms of electronic and partitioning parameters	84

(107). Others have used the products of hydrophobic and electronic parameters. For example, πF, the product of the Hansch-Fujita hydrophobic parameter and the molar attraction constant has been used (112). Similarly, the use of ε log P (33), log Pσ*, and log σ* log P (84) has also been suggested.

In selecting physicochemical parameters to be used in QSAR correlations, one must be conscious of the possibility that those parameters may be mutually dependent. For example, one may find correlations between various pairs of π, σ, E_S, molecular volume, etc. Craig has studied this interdependence and prepared very useful diagrams to aid the investigator in selecting proper combinations of parameters, for example, σ and π (153).

These diagrams are reproduced in Figures 3.1, 3.2, and 3.3.

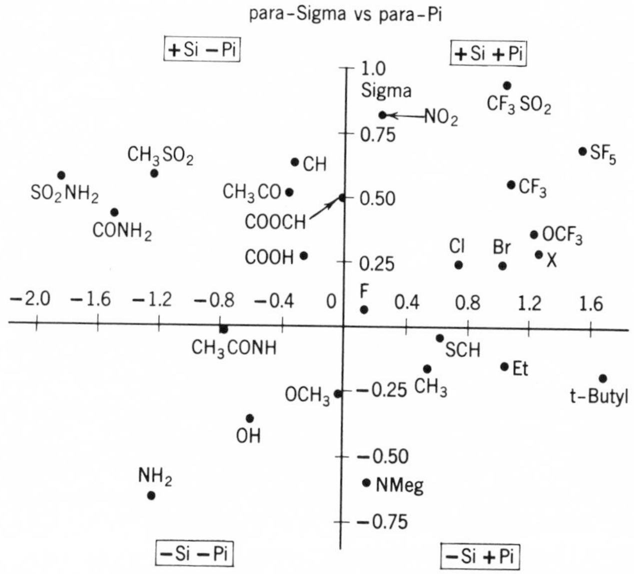

Figure 3.1. Relationship between para-Sigma and para-Pi values.

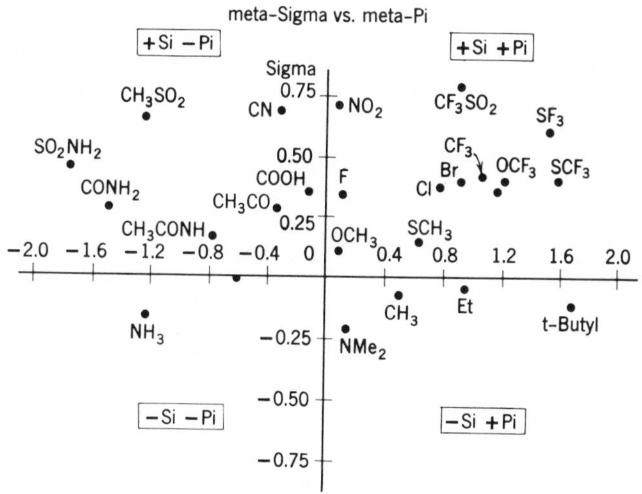

Figure 3.2. Relationship between meta-Sigma and meta-Pi values.

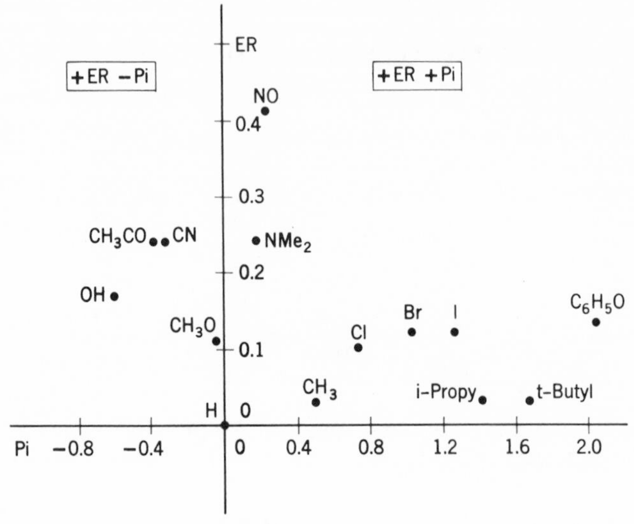

Figure 3.3. Relationship between E_R and Pi values.

In view of the number and nature of the parameters used in the LFER model, it is a just suspicion that many of these parameters are interrelated. Leo and co-workers have recently compared the parameters used and suggested many such relationships (113). In addition, Shorter has addressed the problem of the separation of polar, steric, and resonance effects (154). Indeed, the selection of the parameters to be used in a particular analysis may be a difficult process in view of the complex nature of drug receptor interactions. Also, one should remember that the experimentally determined physicochemical parameters are only an approximation of the factors involved in the biological process.

During the time this book was being written, two excellent review articles (155,156) were published by Hansch and co-workers on partition coefficients and their uses. One of them (155) contains a table of almost 6000 compounds and their log P values along with references to the original measurements. These tables are most valuabl and helpful to one applying the LFER model. Although log P = $\Sigma\pi_i$ has been found to be a reasonable approximation in many systems, there are exceptions where the approximation breaks down rather badly. Therefore, log P is the parameter of choice when it is available from the literature or convenient to measure.

NON-MATHEMATICAL APPLICATION OF THE HANSCH METHOD IN DRUG DESIGN

Frequently in the course of drug design, one is faced with the problem of attempting to maximize a particular type of response in a series of substituted benzenes or benzenoid fused ring systems. When six to twelve compounds in the series are readily available or easily synthesized, the biological response data obtained from these congeners may be subjected to the Hansch-type analysis. From this analysis, although it is not a highly reliable one because it has so few points, the important physicochemical properties necessary for increased activity may be deduced for the compounds. By optimizing these values, one is in a better position to select the most promising compounds for further synthesis and testing.

On the other hand, when the compounds of a series of interest are more difficult to synthesize and when synthesis is considerably more time-consuming than the determination of biological response, the Hansch-type analysis is not always appropriate. In this situation, it is certainly highly desirable to maximize the activity while synthesizing as few compounds as possible. Thus, it would be beneficial to use some rational method for guidance in selecting the most promising succeeding compound for synthesis following the biological study of each individual compound. Recognizing this, Topliss (157) has suggested the use of a non-mathematical operational scheme for analog synthesis. While this method does not utilize the multiple regression analysis, it is still based on the assumptions of the Hansch-type analysis. That is, the idea is based on a qualitative or semi-quantitative selection of the combination of physicochemical properties (π, σ, and E_s) of the particular substituent group in order to maximize the pharmacological activity. Perhaps the best illustration of the method is given in the example operational scheme reported by Topliss in his original paper (157).

In the problem of maximizing the biological activity of a series of aromatic derivatives by first synthesizing and screening the unsubstituted compound, an operational scheme such as that given in Figure 3.4 might be devised.

"Since many systems are $+\pi$ dependent, i.e., activity increases with increasing π values, the p-chloro analog is a good first choice particularly since the ease of synthesis, relative to other substituted phenyl compounds,

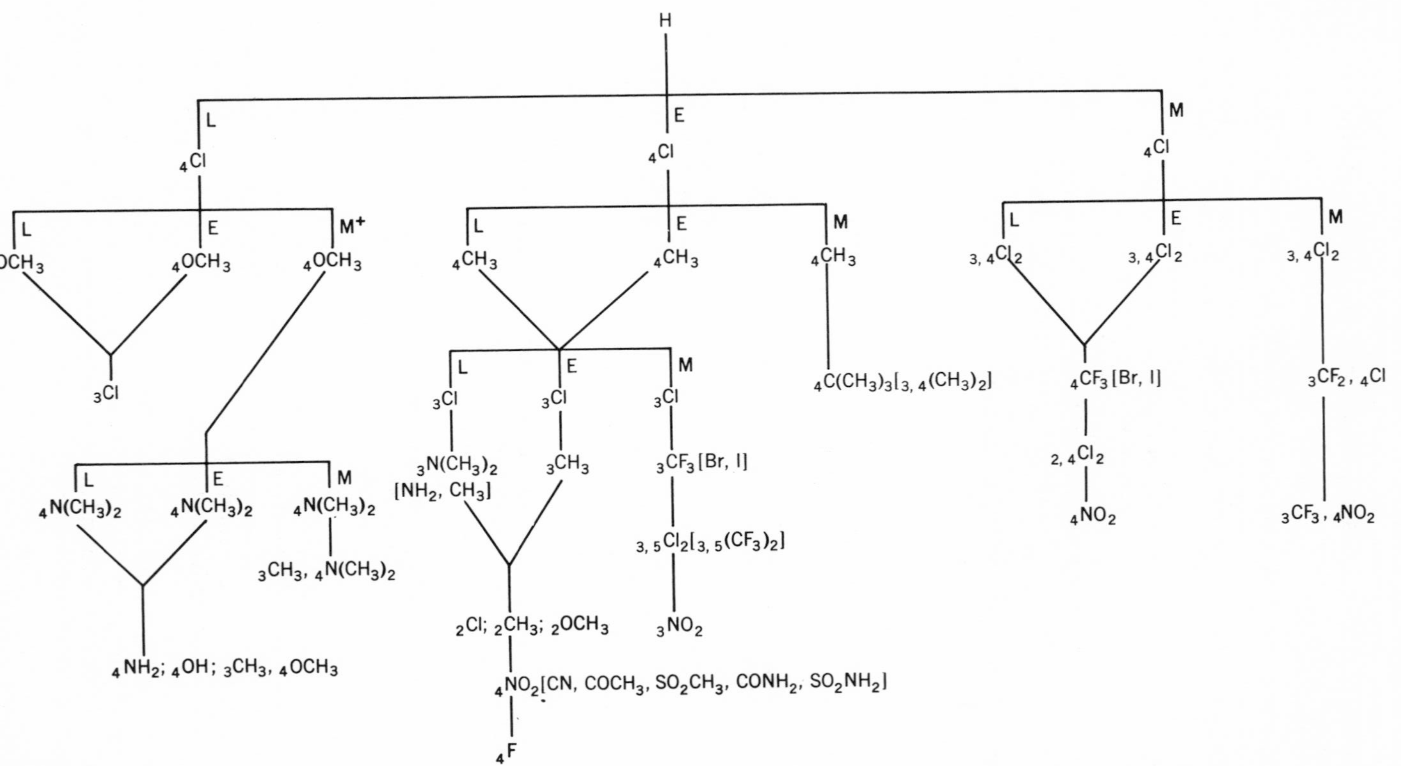

Figure 3.4. Operational scheme for aromatic substitution.

is generally favorable. For the purposes of this analysis, the potency of the 4-chloro compound can be classified as greater than (M), equal to (E), or less than (L) the activity of the parent compound. If the potency is increased, this can be attributed most probably to a $+\pi$ effect, a $+\sigma$ effect (activity increases with increasing σ values) or to a combination of $+\pi$ and $+\sigma$. In this event, the 3,4-dichloro compound would be selected for synthesis next since this would result in both larger $+\pi$ and $+\sigma$ values when summed for the two substituents. Again this particular substituent combination should be highly favorable from a synthetic standpoint. Moving to the stage where the compound has been synthesized and tested, the compound can be classified as more potent, equipotent, or less potent than the 4-chloro analog. If, as seemed most probably, potency did increase, then the 3-CF_3, 4-Cl analog would be the next choice for synthesis since again both $\Sigma\pi$ and $\Sigma\sigma$ would be larger. Assuming again a favorable outcome it would be desirable at this stage to proceed to the 3-CF_3, 4-NO_2 compound since if activity was principally $+\sigma$ controlled a further substantial enhancement of potency should result.

"If, however, the potency of the 3,4-dichloro compound turned out to be about the same as that of the 4-chloro compound, this might be ascribed to either an unfavorable steric effect of meta substitution or to exceeding the optimum lipophilic value of the substituents. In either event the 4-CF_3 analog would then be a good candidate since there is no meta substitution and it would be less lipophilic than the 3,4-dichloro compound but more lipophilic than the 4-Cl compound. Essentially the same arguments can be applied when the 3,4-dichloro analog is less potent than the 4-chloro analog. The 4-bromo and 4-iodo compounds represent alternates to the 4-CF_3 compound. The 2,4-Cl_2 analog might prove interesting particularly if a meta steric effect adversely affected the activity of the 3,4-dichloro analog. The 2,4-isomer should also be slightly less lipophilic than the 3,4-isomer. At the next stage in the sequence the 4-NO_2 should be checked since this could enhance potency if there is an important $+\sigma$ dependency and an optimum π value less than that for the CF_3 group.

"Returning now to the first analog synthesized, the 4-chloro compound, in the event this was found to be about equipotent with the parent compound it could be reasoned that this most probably results from a favorable

$+\pi$ effect counterbalanced by an unfavorable $-\sigma$ dependency. If this is correct, then the 4-CH_3 analog should show enhanced potency since this is a $+\pi-\sigma$ type substituent. Assuming a favorable result the next selection would be the 4-$C(CH_3)_3$ compound with increased $+\pi$ and $-\sigma$ values. An alternate here would be the 3,4-$(CH_3)_2$ analog which might prove advantageous if the high steric requirement of the $C(CH_3)_3$ proved to be a significant negative factor.

"In the situation where the 4-CH_3 compound is equi or less potent than the 4-Cl compound it would seem reasonable to assume either an unfavorable steric effect from para-substitution or a $-\pi$ effect. Since $-\pi$ effects, i.e. decreasing activity with increasing π values are uncommon, the steric explanation seems more probable, hence the next move to 3-Cl in the operational scheme. Assuming that activity increases with this substituent then a sequence is followed, essentially analogous in choice of substituents and reasoning, with that commencing with the 4-CF_3 compound (already discussed) and located on the right hand side of the chart. On the other hand if there is no change in activity with this substituent this could be ascribed to a $+\pi-\sigma$ effect which points to 3-methyl as the next substituent choice. If there is still no potency enhancement the next step would be to examine 2-substituents, chloro, methyl and methoxy. Lack of success in this direction now would prompt the synthesis of the 4-NO_2 analog on the premise that a $+\sigma$ effect is operating but that something less than the π value for Cl is optimal. It will be noted that this is a basically opposite premise from the $+\pi-\sigma$ concept with which the analysis of this central part of the chart commenced. The relative orders of these in the sequence represents a judgement of relative probabilities. Alternatives to 4-NO_2 are 4-CN, $COCH_3$, CH_3SO_2, $COHN_2$ and SO_2NH_2. Assuming that this direction proves favorable there is a good chance that one of these substituents will provide the optimal $+\sigma$, π balance. The remaining choice in the sequence for this branch of the scheme is the 4-F analog which provides the minimal change in π and σ effects compared to the unsubstituted compound. This should prove advantageous in the event that the latter is essentially optimal in terms of π and σ but is subject to rather rapid metabolic transformation by 4-hydroxylation. Returning at this point to the 3-Cl analog, if the potency of this is less than the 4-CH_3 compound which would be consistent with a dominant $-\sigma$ effect the next substituent choice would be 3-$N(CH_3)_2$ (with 3-NH_2 and 3-CH_3 as alternatives).

"The remaining segment of the scheme is concerned with the synthetic sequence to be followed in the case where the 4-chloro analog was found to be significantly less potent than the parent compound. One may conclude that either there is an unfavorable effect from any kind of para substitution for steric reasons, or activity is $-\sigma$ or $-\pi$ controlled. Assuming that the $-\sigma$ effect is the most probable explanation the 4-OCH_3 analog ought to be a favorable selection for synthesis. Confirmation of this in the form of increased activity for the 4-OCH_3 compound would lead to the next choice of the 4-$N(CH_3)_2$ analog where there would be an even greater $-\sigma$ effect. A further trend in the right direction would prompt the synthesis of the 3CH_3, 4$N(CH_3)_2$ compound where the $-\sigma$ effect would be further reinforced. No improvement, or a drop in activity for the $N(CH_3)_2$ analog would perhaps signal some $-\pi$ effect which would suggest synthesis of the 4-NH_2 and 4-OH compounds. The synthesis of the 3-CH_3, 4-OCH_3 analog would be desirable at this stage in the event that the basic character of the 4-$N(CH_3)_2$ function proved to be a negative factor either through ionization or a change in receptor site interaction. Returning to the 4-OCH_3 compound, if this has the same or less activity than the 4-Cl analog, this would indicate unfavorable prospects for para substitution in general and would suggest the synthesis of the 3-Cl compound as the next step. Subsequently, the sequence would proceed as for the 3-Cl compound in the center branch of the chart.

"A similar operational scheme may be drawn up for side chain problems (Figure 3.5). This type of situation arises when groups adjacent to a carbonyl, amino or amide function, for example, are varied. Such situations may be represented by

$$-\overset{\displaystyle O}{\overset{\|}{C}}-R,\ -NHR,\ -\overset{\displaystyle O}{\overset{\|}{C}}-NHR,\ -NH\overset{\displaystyle O}{\overset{\|}{C}}-R$$

where R is the variable substituent. Many other types may, of course, be described. By and large the cases covered are all those other than direct substitution on an aromatic nucleus. Starting with methyl (chart II) as the base compound, the isopropyl substituent would be a good first choice on the premise that a $+\pi$ effect is most probable. Assuming an increase of activity is obtained, cyclopentyl would be the next selection on account of its larger π value with minimal change in E_s, the steric factor. Specific regional hydrophobic bonding is often a positive factor in drug activity while steric

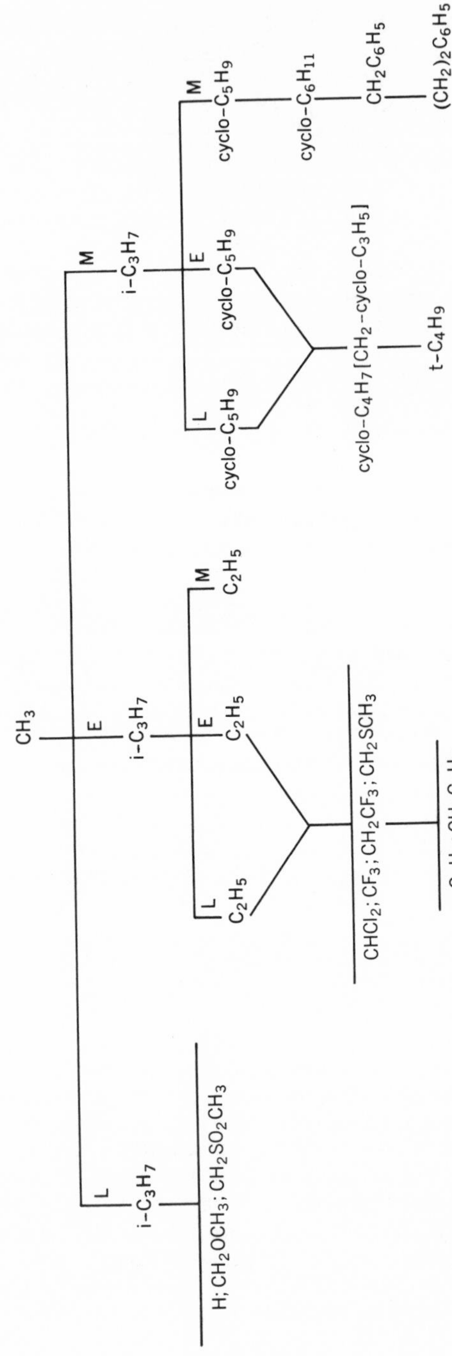

Figure 3.5. Operational scheme for side chains.

requirements if exceeded may prove to be a negative factor. Cycloalkyl groups have the advantage of maximizing the possibility of hydrophobic bonding while minimizing unfavorable steric influences. If enhanced potency is noted with the cyclopentyl compound, the cyclohexyl, benzyl and phenethyl analogs, in sequence, would be prime candidates for synthesis with their progressively larger π values and moderate E_s values. The failure of cyclopentyl to show a potency increases would indicate that the optimum π value had been exceeded thus suggesting cyclobutyl which has the advantage of a very low E_s value in addition to having about the right π value. A suitable alternative choice would be cyclopropylmethyl. A second possibility is that activity is increasing with increasing $-\sigma^*$ values and π is not that important in which case t-butyl should be a favorable substituent.

"Returning now to further consideration of the isopropyl substituent, if there is no potency increase over methyl, it is likely that the π value for maximum activity corresponds to ethyl so that synthesis of the ethyl analog is prompted. If potency decreases or stays the same with ethyl, it could result from an adverse electronic effect which suggests examination of the dichloromethyl, trifluoromethyl, trifluoroethyl and methylthiomethyl substituents which all have $+\sigma^*$ values. As a subsequent step it would be desirable to check the phenyl and benzyl substituents which have higher π values and electronic effects in the desired direction of electron withdrawal relative to ethyl.

"A loss of potency with the isopropyl relative to the methyl substituent would suggest that either the π or σ^* or perhaps both of these values were trending in the wrong direction. In this event the hydrogen, methoxymethyl and methylsulfonylmethyl analogs would be favored elections for further synthetic effort."

To illustrate the practical utility of such operational schemes, Topliss has applied them to several examples from the literature. He found that by applying these schemes the most potent compounds in series consisting of several derivatives would have been arrived at very early in the procedure. These would then be identified quickly for secondary testing thus enhancing the rate of development of a potentially new drug.

Topliss has stressed that these operational schemes presented here are not unique but that other such schemes can be devised to include numerous other substituent groups. These particular schemes merely illustrate the idea. While this method does add another useful tool for the medicinal chemist, the same general procedural and interpretational precautions which apply to the Hansc method should be exercised.

REFERENCES

1. J. M. Clayton, O. E. Millner, Jr., and W. P. Purcell, Ann. Rept. Med. Chem. 1969, 285 (1970).
2. C. Hansch, Intra-Science Chemistry Reports 4, 257 (1970).
3. C. Hansch, Il Farmaco, Ed. Sc 23, 293 (1968).
4. C. Hansch, Proc. 3rd Int. Pharmacol. Meet. 7, 141 (1968).
5. C. Hansch, Accts. Chem. Res. 2, 232 (1969).
6. C. Hansch, Ann. Repts, Med. Chem. 1966, 347 (1967).
7. T. Higuchi and S. S. Davis, J. Pharm. Sci. 59, 1376 (1970).
8. W. P. Purcell and J. M. Clayton, Ann. Repts Med. Chem. 1968, 314 (1969).
9. W. P. Purcell, J. A. Singer, K. Sundaram, and G. L. Parks, "Quantitative Structure-Activity Relationships and Molecular Orbitals in Medicinal Chemistry," in Medicinal Chemistry, 3rd ed., Chapter 10, A. Burger, Ed., John Wiley and Sons, Inc., New York, 1970.
10. C. Hansch in Drug Design, Vol. I, E. J. Ariens, Ed., Academic Press, Inc., New York, in press.
11. C. Hansch and T. Fujita, J. Amer. Chem. Soc. 86, 1616 (1964).
12. C. Hansch, R. M. Muir, T. Fujita, P. P. Maloney, F. Geiger, and M. Streich, J. Amer. Chem. Soc. 85, 2817 (1963).
13. E. Coats, W. R. Glave, and C. Hansch, J. Med. Chem. 13, 913 (1970).
14. E. W. Deutsch and C. Hansch, Nature 211, 75 (1966).
15. T. Fujita and C. Hansch, J. Med. Chem. 10, 991 (1967).
16. T. Fujita, J. Iwasa, and C. Hansch, J. Amer. Chem. Soc. 86, 5175 (1964).
17. C. Hansch, J. Med. Chem. 13, 964 (1970).
18. C. Hansch, J. Org. Chem. 35, 620 (1970).
19. C. Hansch, J. Med. Chem. 11, 920 (1968).
20. C. Hansch and S. M. Anderson, J. Org. Chem. 32, 2583 (1967).
21. C. Hansch and E. W. Deutsch, Biochim. Biophys. Acta 112, 381 (1966).
22. C. Hansch and E. W. Deutsch, J. Med. Chem. 8, 705 (1965).
23. C. Hansch and K. N. Von Kaulla, Biochem. Pharmacol. 19, 2193 (1970).
24. C. Hansch and E. Coats, J. Pharm. Sci. 59, 731 (1970).

25. C. Hansch and R. Kerley, J. Med. Chem. 13, 957 (1970).
26. C. Hansch and F. Helmer, J. Polymer Sci., Part A-1, 6, 3295 (1968).
27. C. Hansch and E. J. Lien, Biochem. Pharmacol. 17, 709 (1968).
28. C. Hansch and E. W. Deutsch, Biochim. Biophys. Acta 126, 117 (1966).
29. C. Hansch and A. R. Steward, J. Med. Chem. 7, 691 (1964).
30. C. Hansch, E. W. Deutsch, and R. N. Smith, J. Amer. Chem. Soc. 87, 2738 (1965).
31. C. Hansch, K. Kiehs, and G. L. Lawrence, J. Amer. Chem. Soc. 87, 5770 (1965).
32. C. Hansch, A. R. Steward, and J. Iwasa, Mol. Pharmacol. 1, 87 (1965).
33. C. Hansch, E. J. Lien, and F. Helmer, Arch. Biochem. Biophys. 128, 319 (1968).
34. C. Hansch, E. Kutter, and A. Leo, J. Med. Chem. 12, 746 (1969).
35. C. Hansch, A. R. Steward, J. Iwasa, and E. W. Deutsch, Mol. Pharmacol. 1, 205 (1965).
36. F. Helmer, K. Kiehs, and C. Hansch, Biochemistry 1 2858 (1968).
37. J. Iwasa, T. Fujita, and C. Hansch, J. Med. Chem. 8, 150 (1965).
38. E. Kutter and C. Hansch, Arch. Biochem. Biophys. 135, 126 (1969).
39. E. Kutter and C. Hansch, J. Med. Chem. 12, 647 (1969).
40. E. J. Lien, C. Hansch, and S. M. Anderson, J. Med. Chem. 11, 430 (1968).
41. E. Miller and C. Hansch, J. Pharm. Sci. 56, 92 (1967).
42. J. Green and S. Marcinkiewicz, J. Chromatogr. 10, 389 (1963).
43. R. W. Taft in Steric Effects in Organic Chemistry, M. S. Newman, Ed., p. 556, John Wiley and Sons, Inc., New York, 1956.
44. C. Hansch. Ann. Repts. Med. Chem. 1967, 348 (1968)
45. O. Exner, Coll. Czech Chem. Commun. 32, 1 (1967).
46. A. Cammarata, S. J. Yau, J. H. Collett, and A. N. Martin, Mol. Pharmacol. 6, 61 (1970).
47. A. Cammarata and S. J. Yau, J. Med. Chem. 13, 93 (1970).
48. K. Bowden and R. C. Young, J. Med. Chem. 13, 225 (1970).
49. M. Charton, J. Amer. Chem. Soc. 91, 615 (1969).

50. R. W. Fuller, M. M. Marsh, and J. Mills, J. Med. Chem. 11, 397 (1968).
51. R. C. Allen, G. L. Carlson, and C. J. Cavallito, J. Med. Chem. 13, 909 (1970).
52. A. E. Bird and A. C. Marshall, Biochem. Pharmacol. 16, 2275 (1967).
53. K. H. Büchel, W. Draber, A. Trebst, and E. Pistorius, Zeit. Naturforsch. 21, 243 (1966).
54. A. Cammarata, J. Med. Chem. 10, 525 (1967).
55. A. Cammarata, J. Med. Chem. 12, 314 (1969).
56. J. M. Clayton and W. P. Purcell, J. Med. Chem. 12, 1087 (1969).
57. D. J. Currie, C. E. Lough, R. F. Silver, and H. L. Holmes, Can. J. Chem. 44, 1035 (1966).
58. T. Fujita, J. Med. Chem. 9, 797 (1966).
59. T. R. Fukuto, R. L. Metcalf, R. L. Jones, and R. O. Myers, J. Agr. Food Chem. 17, 923 (1969).
60. E. R. Garrett, O. K. Wright, G. H. Miller, and K. L. Smith, J. Med. Chem. 9, 203 (1966).
61. H. C. Hemker, Biochim. Biophys. Acta 63, 46 (1962).
62. R. B. Hermann, H. W. Culp, R. E. McMahon, and M. M. Marsh, J. Med. Chem. 12, 749 (1969).
63. R. L. Jones, R. L. Metcalf, and T. R. Fukuto, J. Econ. Entomol. 62, 801 (1969).
64. E. C. Jorgensen and J. W. Reid, J. Med. Chem. 8, 533 (1965).
65. E. C. Jorgensen, R. O. Mulhauser, and R. A. Wilay, J. Med. Chem. 12, 689 (1969).
66. N. Kakeya, N. Yata, A. Kamada, and M. Aoki, Chem. Pharm. Bull. 18, 191 (1970).
67. N. Kakeya, N. Yata, A. Kamada, and M. Aoki, Chem. Pharm. Bull. 17, 2558 (1969).
68. E. J. Lien, M. Hussain, and G. L. Tong, J. Pharm. Sci. 59, 865 (1970).
69. E. J. Lien, M. Hussain, and P. Golden, J. Med. Chem. 13, 623 (1970).
70. R. J. Lukens and J. G. Horsfall, Phytopathology 58, 1671 (1968).
71. Y. C. Martin, J. Med. Chem. 13, 145 (1970).
72. W. B. Neely, H. C. White, and A. Rudzik, J. Pharm. Sci. 57, 1176 (1968).
73. W. B. Neely, W. E. Allison, W. B. Crummett, K. Kauer, and W. Reifschneider, J. Agr. Food. Chem. 18, 45 (1970).
74. P. Pratesi, L. Villa, and E. Grana, Il Farmaco, Ed. Sci. 21, 409 (1966).
75. P. Pratesi, Proc. 3rd Int. Congress Pharmacol. 7, (1968).

76. Y. Sasaki and M. Suzuki, Chem. Pharm. Bull. 17, 1569 (1969).
77. H. J. Schaeffer, R. N. Johnson, E. Odin, and C. Hansch, J. Med. Chem. 13, 452 (1970).
78. M. Tute, J. Med. Chem. 13, 48 (1970).
79. M. Yamazaki, N. Kakeya, T. Morishita, A. Kamada, and M. Aoki, Chem. Pharm. Bull. 18, 708 (1970).
80. P. Bracha and R. D. O'Brien, J. Econ. Entomol. 59, 1255 (1966).
81. A. Cammarata and R. L. Stein, J. Med. Chem. 11, 829 (1968).
82. E. R. Garrett, J. B. Mielck, J. K. Seydel, and H. J Kessler, J. Med. Chem. 12, 740 (1969).
83. G. H. Hamor and E. J. Lien, Il Farmaco, Ed. Sci. 24 704 (1969).
84. C. Hansch and S. M. Anderson, J. Med. Chem. 10, 745 (1967).
85. C. Hansch, A. R. Steward, and J. Iwasa, J. Med. Che 8, 868 (1965).
86. C. Hansch, J. E. Quinlan, and G. L. Lawrence, J. Org. Chem. 33, 347 (1968).
87. C. Hansch, A. R. Steward, S. M. Anderson, and D. Bentley, J. Med. Chem. 11, 1 (1968).
88. M. H. Hussain and E. J. Lien, J. Med. Chem. 14, 138 (1971).
89. K. Kiehs, C. Hansch, and L. Moore, Biochemistry 5, 2602 (1966).
90. E. Kutter, A. Herz, H. J. Teschemacher, and R. Hess J. Med. Chem. 13, 801 (1970).
91. E. J. Lien, J. Med. Chem. 13, 1189 (1970).
92. E. J. Lien, Am. J. Pharm. Educ. 33, 368 (1969).
93. E. J. Lien and C. Hansch, J. Pharm. Sci. 57, 1027 (1968).
94. E. J. Lien, J. Agr. Food Chem. 17, 1265 (1969).
95. B. V. Milborrow and D. A. Williams, Physio. Plant 21, 902 (1968).
96. J. T. Penniston, L. Beckett, D. L. Bentley, and C. Hansch, Mol. Pharmacol. 4, 333 (1969).
97. K. E. Rogers and A. Cammarata, J. Med. Chem. 12, 692 (1969).
98. K. E. Rogers, Proc. Soc. Exp. Biol. Med. 130, 1140 (1969).
99. H. W. Smith, J. Phys. Chem. 25, 605 (1921).
100. H. W. Smith, J. Phys. Chem. 25, 204 (1921).
101. L. S. Bark and R. J. T. Graham, Talanta 13, 1281 (1966).
102. L. S. Bark and R. J. T. Graham, J. Chromatog. 23, 417 (1966).

103. G. L. Biagi, M. C. Guerra, A. M. Barbaro, and M. F. Gamba, J. Med. Chem. 13, 511 (1970).
104. G. L. Biagi, M. C. Guerra, and A. M. Barbaro, Il Farmaco, Ed. Sci. 25, 755 (1970).
105. G. L. Biagi, A. M. Barbaro, and M. C. Guerra, Il Farmaco, Ed. Sc. 25, 749 (1970).
106. C. B. C. Boyce and B. V. Milborrow, Nature 208, 537 (1965).
107. N. J. Turner and R. D. Battershell, Contrib. Boyce Thompson Inst. 24, 139 (1969).
108. J. Halmekoski and A. Nissema, Suomen Kemistilehti B 35, 188 (1962).
109. M. L. Bender, R. L. Van Etten, G. A. Clowes, and J. F. Sebastian, J. Amer. Chem. Soc. 88,2318 (1966).
110. J. H. Hildebrand and R. L. Scott, The Solubility of Non-Electrolytes, 3rd ed., p. 129, Dover Publications, New York, 1964.
111. L. J. Mullins, Chem. Rev. 54, 289 (1954).
112. J. A. Ostrenga, J. Med. Chem. 12, 349 (1969).
113. A. Leo, C. Hansch, and C. Church, J. Med. Chem. 12, 766 (1969).
114. J. C. McGowan, J. Appl. Chem. 1, 1205 (1951).
115. J. C. McGowan, J. Appl. Chem. 4, 41 (1954).
116. J. C. McGowan, Nature 200, 1317 (1963).
117. J. C. McGowan, J. Appl. Chem. 16, 103 (1966).
118. J. C. McGowan, Rec. Trav. Chim. Pays-Bas. 75, 193 (1965).
119. T. R. Fukuto, Residue Reviews 25, 327 (1969).
120. J. J. Zimmerman and J. E. Goyan, J. Med. Chem. 13, 492 (1970).
121. P. N. Craig, H. C. Caldwell, and W. G. Groves, J. Med. Chem. 13, 1079 (1970).
122. C. Hansch and R. Kerley, Chem. Ind., (London) 294, 1969.
123. N. Kakeya, M. Aoki, A. Kamada, and N. Yata, Chem. Pharm. Bull. 17, 1010 (1969).
124. M. Charton, J. Org. Chem. 29, 1222 (1964).
125. A. Cammarata and S. J. Yau, J. Polymer Sci., Part A-1, 8 , 1303 (1970).
126. L. P. Hammett, Physical Organic Chemistry, McGraw-Hill, New York, 1940.
127. H. H. Jaffé, Chem. Rev. 53, 191 (1953).
128. J. E. Leffler and E. Grunwald, Rates and Equilibria of Organic Reactions, John Wiley and Sons, Inc., New York, 1963.
129. D. H. McDaniel and H. C. Brown, J. Org. Chem. 23, 420 (1958).

130. P. R. Wells, Linear Free Energy Relationships, Academic Press, New York, 1968.
131. Y. Yukawa and Y. Tsumo, J. Chem. Soc. Japan (Pure Chemistry Section) 86, 873 (1965).
132. L. P. Hammett, Chem. Rev. 17, 125 (1935).
133. M. Yoshioka, K. Hamamoto, and T. Kubota, Bull. Chem. Soc. Jap. 35, 1723 (1962).
134. E. J. Lien, Drug Intell. Clin. Pharm. 4, 7 (1970).
135. M. Yamazaki, N. Kakeya, T. Morishita, A. Kamada, and M. Aoki, Chem. Parm. Bull. 18, 702 (1970).
136. E. V. Brown and W. H. Kipp, Cancer Res. 29, 1341 (1969).
137. D. Agin, L. Hersh, and D. Holtzman, Proc. Natl. Acad. Sci. U. S. 53, 952 (1965).
138. W. P. Purcell, J. G. Beasley, R. P. Quintana, and J. A. Singer, J. Med. Chem. 9, 297 (1966).
139. M. S. Tute, J. Med. Chem. 13, 48 (1970).
140. J. W. McFarland, Progress in Drug Research 15, 123 (1971).
141. J. A. Ostrenga and C. Steinmetz, J. Pharm. Sci. 59, 414 (1970).
142. T. Yamamoto and T. Otsu, Chem. Ind. (London), 787 (1967).
143. C. G. Swain and E. C. Lupton, J. Amer. Chem. Soc. 90, 4328 (1968).
144. C. C. Price, J. Polymer Sci. 3, 772 (1948).
145. Y. Sasaki and M. Suzuki, Chem. Pharm. Bull. 18, 1759 (1970).
146. Y. Sasaki and M. Suzuki, Chem. Pharm. Bull. 18, 1774 (1970).
147. A. Cammarata, J. Med. Chem. 11, 1111 (1968).
148. K. E. Rogers and A. Cammarata, Biochim. Biophys. Acta 193, 22 (1969).
149. A. J. Wohl, Mol. Pharmacol. 6, 195 (1970).
150. A. Cammarata in Molecular Orbital Studies in Chemical Pharmacology, L. B. Kier, Ed., p. 156, Springer Verlag, New York, 1970.
151. J. W. McFarland, J. Med. Chem. 13, 1192 (1970).
152. W. P. Purcell in Proceedings of the Conference on Structure and Reactions of DFP Sensitive Enzymes, E. Heilbronn, Ed., p. 97, Research Institute on National Defense, Stockholm, 1967.
153. P. N. Craig, J. Med. Chem. 14, 680 (1971).
154. J. Shorter, Quarterly Rev. 24, 433 (1970).
155. A. Leo, C. Hansch, and D. Elkins, Chem. Reviews 71 525 (1971).
156. C. Hansch and W. J. Dunn, J. Pharm. Sci. 61, 1 (1972).

157. J. Topliss, J. Med. Chem., in press.

CHAPTER IV

LINEAR FREE ENERGY-RELATED MODELS: PROCEDURE AND EXAMPLES

The purpose of this chapter is to guide the reader through a hypothetical example and one literature exampl of the LFER model. It is designed to instruct the reade in the stepwise procedure of the application of this mod A purely hypothetical example will be treated first.

Consider the series of molecules

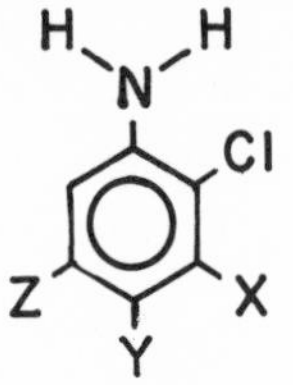

I

where X = H, F, Cl, or Br; Y = H, NO_2, CN, or $COCH_3$; Z = CH_3, C_2H_5, or OCH_3. Therefore, one has 4 X 4 X 4 = 64 possible analogs. Assume that biological activities are available for the derivatives indicated in Table 4.1, an that one wishes to investigate a possible correlation wi π (or preferably log P, if the data are available) and σ from Equation 4.1:

$$\log (1/C) = a \sum_{X,Y,Z} \pi + b \sum_{X,Y,Z} \sigma + c \qquad (4.1$$

C is the molar concentration necessary to give a certain biological response.

Table 4.1 Hypothetical Example, LFER Model Substituent at Position

Cpd.	X^a				Y				Z^a				Log (1/C)
	H	F	Cl	Br	H	NO_2	CN	$COCH_3$	H	CH_3	C_2H_5	OCH_3	
1	X				X				X				3.095
2		X				X			X				6.000
3			X				X				X		5.201
4				X				X				X	5.631
5	X				X							X	3.425
6		X				X					X		5.420
7			X				X			X			5.401
8				X				X	X				5.290

[a]Refer to substituent positions in 1.

Step 1. Determine the sums of π (Table 4.2) and σ (Table 4.2) for each substituent at positions x, y, and z, and substitute these sums in Equation 4.1 to obtain Equations 4.2-4.9 for compounds 1-8, respectively.

$$3.095 = a(0.000) + b(0.000) + c \quad (4.2)$$

$$6.000 = a(0.370) + b(1.115) + c \quad (4.3)$$

$$5.201 = a(1.410) + b(0.963) + c \quad (4.4)$$

$$5.631 = a(0.690) + b(1.008) + c \quad (4.5)$$

$$3.425 = a(0.120) + b(0.115) + c \quad (4.6)$$

$$5.420 = a(1.340) + b(1.045) + c \quad (4.7)$$

$$5.401 = a(0.950) + b(0.964) + c \quad (4.8)$$

$$5.290 = a(0.570) + b(0.893) + c \quad (4.9)$$

Table 4.2 Examples of Hammett σ Values and Hansch π Values[a]

Substituent	σ_m^b	σ_p^b	π_m^c	π_p^c
H	0.000	0.000	0.00	0.0
F	0.337	0.062	0.13	0.1
Cl	0.373	0.227	0.76	0.7
Br	0.391	0.232	0.94	1.0
NO_2	0.710	0.778	0.11	0.2
CN	0.560	0.660	-0.30	-0.3
$COCH_3$	0.376	0.502	-0.28	-0.3
CH_3	-0.069	-0.170	0.51	0.5
C_2H_5	-0.070	-0.151	0.97	
OCH_3	0.115	-0.268	0.12	-0.0

[a]m and p refer to substituents in the meta and para positions, respectively.

[b]Ref. 14

[c]Determined in octanol/water systems for derivatives of phenoxyacetic acid (3).

Step 2. Equations 4.2-4.9 can be solved for the coefficients a and b and the constant c by the method of least squares using one of the several techniques (1). Since biological systems have inherent variations resulting from the experimental evaluations of the activities, one must settle for the "best" set of coefficients (8 equations, 3 unknowns, 5 degrees of freedom). This is a relatively common problem (1) and can be solved "by hand (Appendix II) or by using a computer program (Appendix III) for the solution of a multiple regression analysis.

Step 3. Once the values for a, b, and c are determined, Equation 4.1 becomes Equation 4.10:

$$\log(1/C) = -0.373\Sigma\pi + 2.709\Sigma\sigma + 3.120 \qquad (4.1$$

This is the equation which best fits the hypothetical set of data and corresponding molecular modifications in terms of σ and π. In order to determine if the correlation is meaningful, one must calculate its statistical significance. This requires obtaining the calculated biological activities of the compounds by solution of Equation 4.10 for each congener. For example, the calculated value for compound 2 (Table 4.1) is 6.002 (4.11):

$$\log 1/C = -0.373(0.370) + 2.709(1.115) + 3.120$$

$$= 6.002 \qquad (4.11)$$

Following this procedure for the remainder of the compounds, the values in Table 4.3 are obtained.

As a basis for the statistical significance of the regression, the statistical tests outlined in Chapter II may be used.

Multiple Correlation Coefficient R and R^2 (Chapter II, Equation 2.14)

$$R^2 = \frac{\Sigma(\hat{Y}-\bar{Y})^2}{\Sigma(Y-\bar{Y})^2} = \frac{7.9486}{7.9331} = 1.00 \qquad (4.12)$$

$$R = \sqrt{R^2} = \sqrt{1.00} = 1.00 \qquad (4.13)$$

It should be noted here that the correlation coefficient of 1.00 (representing "perfect" correlation) is highly unusual. Due to the rounding of numbers carried out in the hand calculations, the chances of this occurring are increased in the instances of very good correlations. When the solution of the analysis was carried out on the computer using the program in Appendix III, R^2 was found to be 0.998 and R = 0.998. In addition, it might be noted that the coefficients of the independent variables in the regression equation may vary slightly between the hand computation (Appendix II) and that using the computer program in Appendix III for this same reason.

Significance of the Regression F (Chapter II, Equation 2.15)

Table 4.3 Observed and Calculated Activities for the Hypothetical Example

Compound	Substituents at Position												Log 1/C	
	X[a]				Y				Z[a]					
	H	F	Cl	Br	H	NO_2	CN	$COCH_3$	H	CH_3	C_2H_5	OCH_3	Observed	Calculated[b]
1	X				X				X				3.095	3.120
2		X				X			X				6.000	6.002
3			X				X				X		5.201	5.203
4				X				X				X	5.631	5.593
5	X				X							X	3.425	3.387
6		X				X					X		5.420	5.451
7			X				X			X			5.401	5.377
8				X				X	X				5.390	5.327
P-1		X				X						X		6.269
P-2		X					X					X		6.156
P-3			X			X				X				5.487

[a]Refers to substituent positions in 1.

[b]Calculated using Equation 4.10

$$F = \frac{\Sigma(\hat{Y}-Y)^2/(k-1)}{\Sigma(Y-\hat{Y})^2/(n-k)} = \frac{(7.9486)/(3-1)}{(0.0064)/(8-3)} = 3104.9 \qquad (4.14)$$

$F_{(k,n-k-1)} = F_{(2,5)} = 37.1$ at the 99.9 confidence level.

Explained Variance EV
(Chapter II, Equation 2.16)

$$E.V. = 1 - \frac{\Sigma(\hat{Y}-Y)^2/(n-k)}{\Sigma(Y-\overline{Y})^2/(n-1)} = \frac{(0.0064)/(8-3)}{(7.933)/(8-1)} = 0.9989 \quad (4.15)$$

As a result of these tests and in view of the discussion of statistical significance in Chapter II, one is allowed to say that the biological data of our hypothetical example exhibits a high degree of correlation (at the 99% confidence level) with the physicochemical parameters π and σ.

Step 4. As was suggested earlier, one of the reasons for subjecting biological data to a regression analysis is to "expand" the data to molecules which have not been tested (and possibly not synthesized) in order to suggest more promising molecules for further investigation. As was pointed out in Step 1, there are a possible 64 total congeners in our series of 4 different substituent groups at each of 3 substituent positions. Since only 8 compounds were subjected to the analysis, we are able to assign a "predicted" activity value (log 1/C) to the remaining 56 congeners. This is achieved mechanically by resubstitution of the π and σ values of the substituent groups of the compound into the regression equation (4.10).

For example, we could "predict" the activity of the compound containing substituent groups, F, NO_2, and CN (P-1, Table 4.3) at positions X, Y, and Z, respectively. The resulting equation yields a response parameter of 6.269--a greater activity value than that of any of the compounds actually tested. Similarly compound P-2 (Table 4.3) also has a greater predicted activity than that of any of those compounds tested. On the other hand, compound P-3 (Table 4.3) exhibits a higher calculated activity than most of those congeners tested but less than the most active evaluated compounds. By this same process, the activities of the remaining 53 compounds in the series may be calculated, and this may suggest some guidelines for more productive synthesis and evaluation.

The hypothetical example was introduced to illustrate the procedure and mechanism of applying the LFER model. Consider now a "real-life" example.

In 1963, Graham and Kamar studied the adrenergic blocking activity of a series of β-haloalkylamines (2). As a result of their study, they reported the ED_{50} values (ED_{50} is defined as the dosage required to elicit a defined effective, therapeutic response in 50% of the population) of 22 N,N-dimethyl-2-bromo-phenethylamines (II) in their antagonism to adrenaline in the rat.

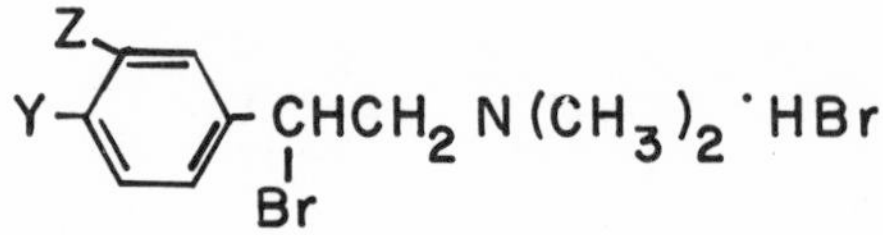

$Y(Z)C_6H_3$–$CH(Br)CH_2N(CH_3)_2 \cdot HBr$

II

In II, Y and Z represent substituent positions on the parent molecule. The reported data are given in Table 4.4. After assuming the data to follow the criteria outlined in Chapter III and inspecting it for "unusual" congeners, the first step is to convert the biological response parameters to their negative logarithms using Equation 4.1. The "new" response data (log 1/C = log 1/molar ED_{50}) is given in Table 4.5. The next step is then the collection of the physicochemical parameters for study. Several extensive collections of physicochemical parameters are easily obtained from the literature. For example, tables of π values (3,4), P values (4-11), σ constants (12-15), σ^* parameters (13,15,16), pK_A values (17), σ_I parameters (13,15), and E_s values (13,16) are readily available. In this particular example previously analyzed by Hansch and Lien, they chose the Hansch-Fujita hydrophobic parameter π and the Hammett electronic parameter σ (18).

The π constants used in this analysis are those derived from a phenoxyacetic acid system measured in octanol and water and reported by Fujita et al. (3). These substituent values are listed in Table 4.6. σ values were obtained from the compilation of Jaffé (19) and are also listed in Table 4.5. The subscripts Y and Z refer to the positions on the parent molecule at which the substituents are located.

Since there is more than one substituent position on the parent molecule in this series, the physicochemical parameters for the two substituent groups in each compound

Table 4.4
Antagonism of N,N-Dimethyl-2-Bromophenethylamines to Adrenaline. I. Biological Data

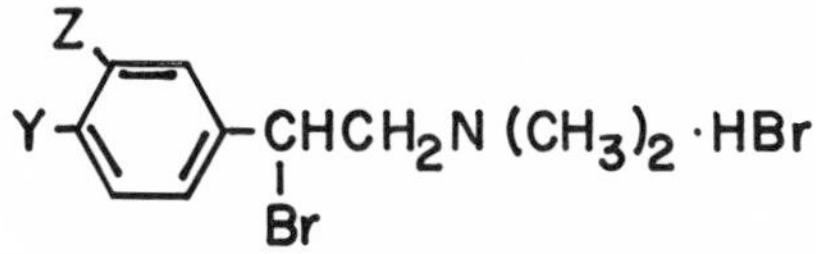

Y-$C_6H_3(Z)$-$CH(Br)CH_2N(CH_3)_2 \cdot HBr$

Compound	Substituent at Y	Substituent at Z	ED_{50}[a]
9	H	H	35.00 ± 7.00
10	F	H	7.00 ± 2.00
11	Cl	H	2.10 ± 0.30
12	Br	H	1.30 ± 0.20
13	I	H	0.56 ± 0.05
14	CH_3	H	0.50 ± 0.05
15	H	F	30.00 ± 6.00
16	H	Cl	7.00 ± 1.40
17	H	Br	5.00 ± 1.20
18	H	I	4.00 ± 0.90
19	H	CH_3	3.50 ± 0.90
20	F	Cl	6.40 ± 1.10
21	F	Br	2.70 ± 0.40
22	F	CH_3	1.50 ± 0.30
23	Cl	Cl	1.30 ± 0.20
24	Cl	Br	1.20 ± 0.06
25	Cl	CH_3	1.10 ± 0.07
26	Br	Cl	1.00 ± 0.01
27	Br	Br	0.45 ± 0.02
28	Br	CH_3	0.60 ± 0.07
29	CH_3	CH_3	0.50 ± 0.04
30	CH_3	Br	0.30 ± 0.01

[a]From (2) in moles X 10^{-9} of body weight.

Table 4.5
Antagonism of N,N-Dimethyl-2-Bromophenethylamines to Adrenaline. II. Substituent Parameters

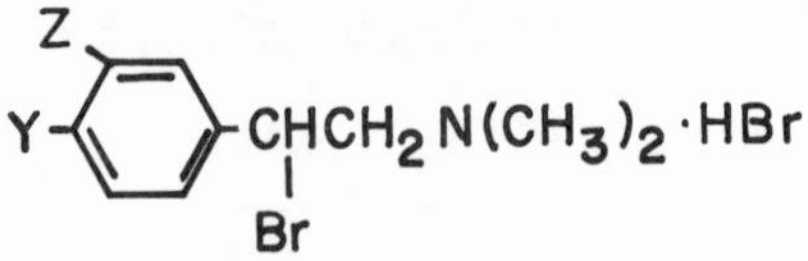

$Y-C_6H_3(Z)-CH(Br)CH_2N(CH_3)_2 \cdot HBr$

Compound	Substituent at						log 1/C[c]
	Y	π_Y[a]	σ_Y[b]	Z	π_Z[a]	σ_Z[b]	
9	H	0.00	0.00	H	0.00	0.00	7.46
10	F	0.15	0.06	H	0.00	0.00	8.16
11	Cl	0.70	0.23	H	0.00	0.00	8.68
12	Br	1.02	0.23	H	0.00	0.00	8.89
13	I	1.26	0.28	H	0.00	0.00	9.25
14	CH_3	0.52	-0.17	H	0.00	0.00	9.30
15	H	0.00	0.00	F	0.13	0.34	7.52
16	H	0.00	0.00	Cl	0.76	0.37	8.16
17	H	0.00	0.00	Br	0.94	0.39	8.30
18	H	0.00	0.00	I	1.15	0.35	8.40
19	H	0.00	0.00	CH_3	0.51	-0.07	8.46
20	F	0.15	0.06	Cl	0.76	0.37	8.19
21	F	0.15	0.06	Br	0.94	0.39	8.57
22	F	0.15	0.06	CH_3	0.51	-0.07	8.82
23	Cl	0.70	0.23	Cl	0.76	0.37	8.89
24	Cl	0.70	0.23	Br	0.94	0.39	8.92
25	Cl	0.70	0.23	CH_3	0.51	-0.07	8.96
26	Br	1.02	0.23	Cl	0.76	0.37	9.00
27	Br	1.02	0.23	Br	0.94	0.39	9.35
28	Br	1.02	0.23	CH_3	0.51	-0.07	9.22
29	CH_3	0.52	-0.17	CH_3	0.51	-0.07	9.30
30	CH_3	0.52	-0.17	Br	0.94	0.39	9.52

[a]From phenoxyacetic acid system, Ref. 3.

[b]Ref. 19.

[c]Ref. 2.

Table 4.6
Antagonism of N,N-Dimethyl-2-Bromophenethylamines to Adrenaline. III. Summation of Substituent Parameters

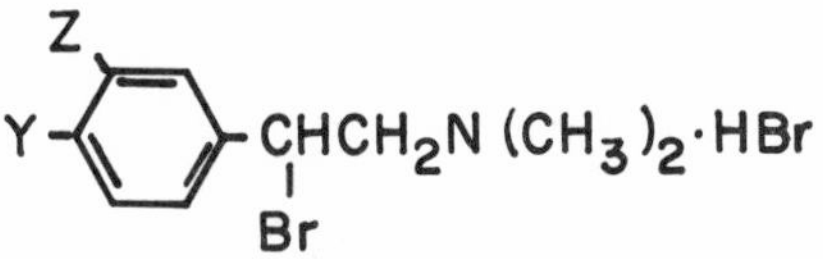

$Y\text{-}C_6H_3(Z)\text{-}CH(Br)CH_2N(CH_3)_2\cdot HBr$

Compound	Substituent at Y	Z	$\Sigma\pi$[a]	$(\Sigma\pi)^2$	$\Sigma\sigma$[b]	log 1/C[c]
9	H	H	0.00	0.00	0.00	7.46
10	F	H	0.15	0.02	0.06	8.16
11	Cl	H	0.70	0.49	0.23	8.68
12	Br	H	1.02	1.04	0.23	8.89
13	I	H	1.26	1.59	0.28	9.25
14	CH_3	H	0.52	0.27	-0.17	9.30
15	H	F	0.13	0.02	0.34	7.52
16	H	Cl	0.76	0.58	0.37	8.16
17	H	Br	0.94	0.88	0.39	8.30
18	H	I	1.15	1.32	0.35	8.40
19	H	CH_3	0.51	0.26	-0.07	8.46
20	F	Cl	0.91	0.83	0.43	8.19
21	F	Br	1.09	1.19	0.45	8.57
22	F	CH_3	0.66	0.44	-0.01	8.82
23	Cl	Cl	1.46	2.13	0.60	8.89
24	Cl	Br	1.64	2.69	0.62	8.92
25	Cl	CH_3	1.21	1.46	0.16	8.96
26	Br	Cl	1.78	3.17	0.60	9.00
27	Br	Br	1.96	3.84	0.62	9.35
28	Br	CH_3	1.53	2.34	0.16	9.22
29	CH_3	CH_3	1.03	1.06	-0.24	9.30
30	CH_3	Br	1.46	2.13	0.22	9.52

[a]Ref. 3.
[b]Ref. 19.
[c]Ref. 2.

must be summed to obtain the overall parameters for the molecule. That is, Equation 3.1 becomes Equation 4.16 for this series:

$$\log 1/C = a\Sigma(\pi_Y + \pi_Z)^2 + b\Sigma(\pi_Y + \pi_Z) + \rho\Sigma(\sigma_Y + \sigma_Z) + c \quad (4.16)$$

It is generally represented by Equation 4.17:

$$\log 1/C = -a(\Sigma\pi)^2 + b\Sigma\pi + \rho\Sigma\sigma + c \quad (4.17)$$

One might recall here that a basic requisite for valid substituent physicochemical parameters for this method is that they be additive. Therefore, for compounds 9, 10, 20, and 22, for example, Equations 4.18, 4.19, 4.20, and 4.21, respectively, may now be generated:

$$\log 1/C = 7.46 = -a\Sigma(\pi_{H_Y} + \pi_{H_Z})^2 + b\Sigma'(\pi_{H_Y} + \pi_{H_Z}) + \rho\Sigma(\sigma_{H_Y} + \sigma_{H_Z}) + c \quad (4.18)$$

$$\log 1/C = 8.16 = -a\Sigma(\pi_{F_Y} + \pi_{H_Z})^2 + b\Sigma(\pi_{F_Y} + \pi_{H_Z}) + \rho\Sigma(\sigma_{F_Y} + \sigma_{H_Z}) + c \quad (4.19)$$

$$\log 1/C = 8.19 = -a\Sigma(\pi_{F_Y} + \pi_{Cl_Z})^2 + b\Sigma(\pi_{F_Y} + \pi_{Cl_Z}) + \rho\Sigma(\sigma_{F_Y} + \sigma_{Cl_Z}) + c \quad (4.20)$$

$$\log 1/C = 8.82 = -a\Sigma(\pi_{F_Y} + \pi_{CH_{3_Z}})^2 + b\Sigma(\pi_{F_Y} + \pi_{CH_{3_Z}}) + \rho\Sigma(\sigma_{F_Y} + \sigma_{CH_{3_Z}}) + c \quad (4.21)$$

Similar equations are then generated for the remainder of the compounds and appropriate parameters are substituted into the equations to generate mathematically meaningful and soluble ones. Thus, in this example when the values for π and σ listed in Table 4.5 are substituted into Equations 4.18-4.21. Equations 4.22-4.25, respectively, are obtained for compounds 9, 10, 20, 22:

$$7.46 = -a(0.00 + 0.00)^2 + b(0.00 + 0.00) + \rho(0.00 + 0.00) + c \quad (4.22)$$

$$8.16 = -a(0.15 + 0.00)^2 + b(0.15 + 0.00) + \rho)0.06 + 0.00) + c \quad (4.23)$$

$$8.19 = -a(0.15 + 0.76)^2 + b(0.15 + 0.76) + \rho(0.06 + 0.37) + c \qquad (4.24)$$

$$8.82 = -a(0.15 + 0.51)^2 + b(0.15 + 0.51) + \rho(0.06 - 0.07) + c \qquad (4.25)$$

Reduction of these equations yields final Equations 4.26-4.29 for compounds 9, 10, 20, and 22, respectively:

$$-a(0.00) + b(0.00) + \rho(0.00) + c = 7.46 \qquad (4.26$$

$$-a(0.02) + b(0.15) + \rho(0.06) + c = 8.16 \qquad (4.27)$$

$$-a(0.83) + b(0.91) + \rho(0.43) + c = 8.19 \qquad (4.28)$$

$$-a(0.44) + b(0.66) + \rho(-0.01) + c = 8.82 \qquad (4.29)$$

Similarly, reduced equations are determined for the remaining 18 compounds. Table 4.6 gives a summary of the terms in these reduced equations. The resulting 22 equations with 4 unknowns (a, b, ρ, and c) are then solved simultaneously by the method of least squares (Appendix III). It might be noted that, unlike the Free-Wilson method (Chapter VI), this method not only allows the inclusion of substituent groups observed only once in a series, but is also conducive to resulting in the very desirable high number of degrees of freedom (in this example, 18) to yield greater statistically significant results (20).

One should also realize that the values obtained thus far do not limit the investigator to one analysis. Rather, the values in this table alone allow analyses according to combinations or modifications of at least Equations 3.1-3.5 (Chapter III). Other equations are also possible.

From the regression analysis of this data, Equation 4.30 was generated to describe the biological activity in terms of the π and σ parameters:

$$\log 1/C = -0.096\pi^2 + 1.387\pi - 1.537\sigma + 7.831 \qquad (4.30)$$

The statistics of the analysis ($R = 0.918$, $R^2 = 0.843$, $EV = 0.817$, $F = 32.29$) indicate that the agreement between the observed and calculated response values is very good. In attempts to delineate the relative importance of the various parameters to the biological response, however, analyses were also made according to Equations 3.3-3.5 (Chapter III). The results of these analyses are given in Equations 4.31-4.33:

$$\log 1/C = 1.226\pi - 1.577\sigma + 7.890 \qquad (4.31)$$

$$\log 1/C = 0.769\pi + 7.932 \qquad (4.32)$$

$$\log 1/C = -0.037\sigma + 8.704 \qquad (4.33)$$

The statistical parameters obtained for these analyses indicate that Equation 4.31 ($R = 0.917$, $R^2 = 0.841$, EV $= 0.824$, $F = 50.10$) describes the biological response much better than do Equation 4.32 ($r = 0.724$, $r^2 = 0.524$, EV $= 0.500$, $F = 22.02$) or Equation 4.33 ($r = 0.022$, $r^2 = 0.000$, EV $= 0.050$, $F = 0.01$). If one compares Equation 4.32 and 4.33, it is apparent that the more important character of the substituent in affecting the biological activity is its hydrophobic bonding ability. Equation 4.31, however, shows that electronic effects do play a significant role in eliciting activity. Furthermore, the role of π appears to be linear since the π^2 term (4.30) does not increase the statistical significance of the regression. Thus, it is concluded that of the equations and parameters used, Equation 4.31 containing linear σ and π terms best describes the response parameter.

The parameters used as a judge of the statistical significance are based upon the differences between the observed activities and those calculated from the regression equations. Following our hypothetical model, the calculated activities are obtained by resolution of the linear equations which comprise the regression analysis employing the constants generated by the regression. For example, for compound 20, Equation 4.34 is resolved using the values for b, ρ, and c from Equation 4.31:

$$\log 1/C = b(0.91) + \rho(0.43) \qquad (4.34)$$

The results are given in Equation 4.35:

$$\log 1/C = 1.221(0.91) - 1.587(0.43) + 7.88 = 8.32 \qquad (4.35)$$

This response value (8.32) differs only slightly from the observed value (8.19). This process is then repeated for the entire series. The results are given in Table 4.7.

An additional value of the final equation lies in its potential use to expand the series of data by suggesting which compounds not included in the study might have the greatest potential as active agents. This is accomplished by simply resolving the regression equation (4.31) using the physicochemical parameters of additional substituents. It might be noted that Equation 4.31

Table 4.7
Antagonism of N,N-Dimethyl-2-Bromophenethylamines to Adrenaline. IV. Observed vs. Calculated Activities

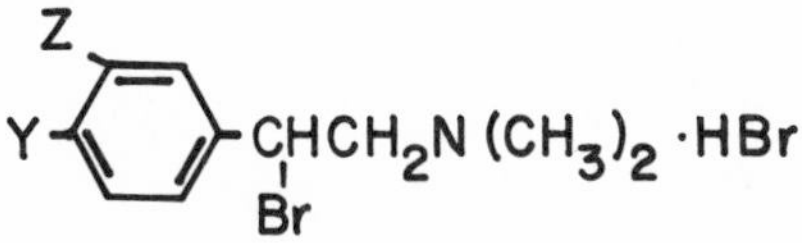

$$\text{Y-}\langle\text{C}_6\text{H}_3(\text{Z})\rangle\text{-CH(Br)CH}_2\text{N(CH}_3)_2 \cdot \text{HBr}$$

Compound	Substituent at X	Substituent at Y	log 1/C Observed[a]	log 1/C Calculated[b]	Δ log 1/C[c]
9	H	H	7.46	7.89	-0.43
10	F	H	8.16	7.98	0.18
11	Cl	H	8.68	8.38	0.30
12	Br	H	8.89	8.77	0.12
13	I	H	9.25	8.98	0.27
14	CH_3	H	9.30	8.79	0.51
15	H	F	7.52	7.51	0.01
16	H	Cl	8.16	8.23	-0.07
17	H	Br	8.30	8.42	-0.12
18	H	I	8.40	8.74	-0.34
19	H	CH_3	8.46	8.62	-0.16
20	F	Cl	8.19	8.32	-0.13
21	F	Br	8.57	8.51	0.06
22	F	CH_3	8.82	8.71	0.11
23	Cl	Cl	8.89	8.72	0.17
24	Cl	Br	8.92	8.91	0.01
25	Cl	CH_3	8.96	9.11	-0.15
26	Br	Cl	9.00	9.11	-0.11
27	Br	Br	9.35	9.30	0.05
28	Br	CH_3	9.22	9.49	-0.27
29	CH_3	CH_3	9.30	9.53	-0.23
30	CH_3	Br	9.52	9.32	0.20
P-4	I	I		9.83	
P-5	I	CH_3		9.72	

[a]Ref. 2.

[b]Calculated using Equation 4.31 (18).

[c]$(\log 1/C)_{obs} - (\log 1/C)_{calc}$.

suggests that substituents with lower positive or negativ σ values and with higher positive π properties would have the greatest activity. Two examples of the predicted activities of compounds (P-4 and P-5) are given in Table 4.7. Their activities were calculated from Equations 4.36 and 4.37, respectively:

$$\log 1/C = 1.221(1.26 + 1.15) - 1.587(0.28 + 0.35) + 7.88 = 9.83 \quad (4.36)$$

$$\log 1/C = 1.221(1.26 + 0.51) - 1.587(0.28 - 0.07) + 7.88 = 9.72 \quad (4.37)$$

Both of these compounds have higher calculated biological response parameters than any of those compounds tested. It should also be noted that the activities of compounds containing substituent groups other than those tested may also be calculated from the regression equation. Extreme caution should be exercised, however, in selecting those substituents which do not differ too drastically in overall properties from those included in the analysis.

EXAMPLE 2

A second literature example is a gross modification of an analysis by Kutter and Hansch (21). In 1968 Fuller et al reported the monoamine oxidase inhibitory potencies of a series of N-(phenoxyethyl)cyclopropylamines (22). Table 4.8 gives the pI_{50} values (negative logarithm of the mola concentration necessary to elicit 50% of the enzyme) of 18 compounds reported.

Since pI_{50} represents log 1/C, no additional attraction of the activity data is necessary. For this particular study the substituent parameters π, E_S, and σ were considered. A summary of the parameters used is given in Table 4.9. Following the procedure outlined in the previous two examples analyses were made using several variations of the generalized Hansch equation. A summary of the generated equations (4.38-4.49) is given in Table 4.10.

Careful study of Equations 4.38-4.49 indicates that the most statistically significant equation is Equation 4.46 in E_s and σ. By comparison of the statistical tests of each equation, one is able to delineate those physicochemical parameters which correlate best with the respons parameter and may thereby indicate their relative importance in eliciting a pharmacological or biochemical

Table 4.8 Cyclopropylamine Inhibitors of Monoamine Oxidase[a]

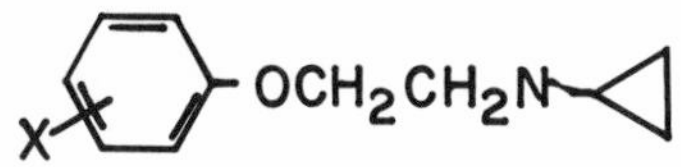

Compound	Substituent at X	log 1/C[a]
31	4-Br	6.64
32	3,4-Cl_2	6.30
33	3-NO_2	5.76
34	3-CF_3	4.98
35	4-CH_3	5.69
36	3,5-Cl_2	5.68
37	3-Cl-4-CH_3	5.75
38	3-Br	5.64
39	3-CH_3-4-Cl	6.06
40	4-Cl	5.82
41	4-OCH_3	5.46
42	3,4-$(CH_3)_2$	4.71
43	3,5-$(CH_3)_2$	4.85
44	3-CH_3	4.78
45	4-Cl-3,5-$(CH_3)_2$	4.70
46	3,4,5-$(CH_3)_3$	3.54
47	4-N=NC_6H_5	7.56
48	4-NH_2	4.40

[a]Ref. 22. pI_{50} values (negative logarithm of the molar concentration of compound necessary to elicit 50% inhibition of the enzyme).

Table 4.9
Substituent Parameters Used in the Analysis of the pI_{50} Values of Selected Cyclopropylamine Monoamine Oxidase Inhibitors

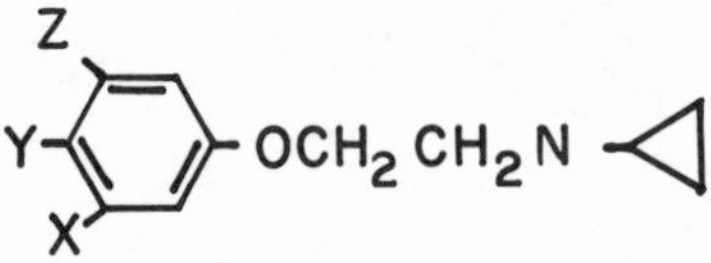

Compound	Substituent at X	y	z	π^a π_x	π_y	π_z	$\Sigma\pi$	$\Sigma\pi^2$
31	H	BR	H	0.00	1.02	0.00	1.02	1.04
32	Cl	Cl	H	0.76	0.70	0.00	1.46	2.13
33	NO_2	H	H	0.11	0.00	0.00	0.11	0.01
34	CF_3	H	H	1.07	0.00	0.00	1.07	1.14
35	H	CH_3	H	0.00	0.52	0.00	0.52	0.27
36	Cl	H	Cl	0.76	0.00	0.76	1.52	2.31
37	Cl	CH_3	H	0.76	0.52	0.00	1.28	1.64
38	Br	H	H	0.94	0.00	0.00	0.94	0.88
39	CH_3	Cl	H	0.51	0.70	0.00	1.21	1.46
40	Cl	H	H	0.76	0.00	0.00	0.76	0.58
41	H	OCH_3	H	0.00	-0.04	0.00	-0.04	0.00
42	CH_3	CH_3	H	0.51	0.52	0.00	1.03	1.06
43	CH_3	H	CH_3	0.51	0.51	0.00	1.02	1.04
44	CH_3	H	H	0.51	0.00	0.00	0.51	0.26
45	CH_3	Cl	CH_3	0.51	0.70	0.51	1.72	2.96
46	CH_3	CH_3	CH_3	0.51	0.52	0.51	1.54	2.92
47	H	$N{=}NC_6H_5$	H	0.00	1.71	0.00	1.71	2.92
48	H	NH_2	H	0.00	-1.63	0.00	-1.63	2.66

[a]From phenoxyacetic acid system (3).
[b]Ref. 21.
[c]Ref. 19.
[d]Ref. 22.

Table 4.9 Continued

Cpd.	E_s^b				σ^c				
	E_s^x	E_s^y	E_s^z	ΣE_s	σ_x	σ_y	σ_z	$\Sigma\sigma$	log 1/C[δ]
31	1.24	0.00	1.24	2.48	0.00	0.23	0.00	0.23	6.64
32	0.27	0.00	1.24	1.51	0.37	0.23	0.00	0.60	6.30
33	-1.28	0.00	1.24	-0.04	0.71	0.00	0.00	0.71	5.76
34	-1.16	0.00	1.24	0.08	0.42	0.00	0.00	0.42	4.98
35	1.24	0.00	1.24	2.48	0.00	-0.17	0.00	-0.17	5.69
36	0.27	0.00	0.27	0.54	0.37	0.00	0.37	0.74	5.68
37	0.27	0.00	1.24	1.51	0.37	-0.17	0.00	0.20	5.75
38	0.08	0.00	1.24	1.32	0.39	0.00	0.00	0.39	5.64
39	0.00	0.00	1.24	1.24	-0.07	0.23	0.00	0.16	6.06
40	0.27	0.00	1.24	1.51	0.37	0.00	0.00	0.37	5.82
41	1.24	0.00	1.24	2.48	0.00	-0.27	0.00	-0.27	5.46
42	0.00	0.00	1.24	1.24	-0.07	-0.17	0.00	-0.24	4.71
43	0.00	0.00	0.00	0.00	-0.07	0.00	-0.07	-0.14	4.85
44	0.00	0.00	1.24	1.24	-0.07	0.00	0.00	-0.07	4.78
45	0.00	0.00	0.00	0.00	-0.07	0.23	-0.07	0.09	4.70
46	0.00	0.00	0.00	0.00	-0.07	-0.17	-0.07	-0.31	3.54
47	1.24	0.00	1.24	2.48	0.00	0.64	0.00	0.64	7.56
48	1.24	0.00	1.24	2.48	0.00	-0.66	0.00	-0.66	4.40

Table 4.10 Equations Generated by Regression Analysis of the Monoamine Oxidase Inhibitory Potencies of Selected Cyclopropylamines

Equation	Standard Statistical Tests					Eq. No.
	R	R^2	EV	F-ratio	s	
$\log 1/C = -0.044\pi^2 + 0.176\pi + 0.676 E_s + 1.698\sigma + 4.269$	0.942	0.889	0.855	26.00	0.350	(4.38)
$\log 1/C = -0.133\pi^2 + 0.645\pi + 0.661 E_s + 4.252$	0.705	0.497	0.390	4.61	0.717	(4.39)
$\log 1/C = -0.022\pi^2 - 0.128\pi + 1.657\sigma + 5.358$	0.672	0.451	0.333	3.84	0.749	(4.40)
$\log 1/C = -0.109\pi^2 + 0.336\pi + 5.318$	0.280	0.078	0.045	0.63	0.938	(4.41)
$\log 1/C = 0.294\pi + 5.205$	0.257	0.066	0.008	1.13	0.914	(4.42)
$\log 1/C = 0.154\pi + 0.674E_s + 1.716\sigma + 4.226$	0.942	0.887	0.863	36.59	0.340	(4.43)
$\log 1/C = 0.591\pi + 0.656E_s + 4.123$	0.692	0.479	0.410	6.89	0.705	(4.44)
$\log 1/C = -0.139\pi + 1.666\sigma + 5.335$	0.671	0.451	0.378	6.15	0.724	(4.45)
$\log 1/C = 0.639E_s + 1.858\sigma + 4.384$	0.935	0.875	0.858	52.49	0.345	(4.46)
$\log 1/C = 0.472E_s + 4.870$	0.499	0.249	0.202	5.30	0.820	(4.47)
$\log 1/C = 1.520\sigma + 5.235$	0.663	0.440	0.405	12.57	0.708	(4.48)
$\log 1/C = 0.023\pi^2 + 5.493$	0.024	0.001	0.062	0.01	0.945	(4.49)

Table 4.11 Inhibitors of Monoamine Oxidase. Observed vs. Calculated Activities

$$\text{3-X, 4-Y, 5-Z-C}_6\text{H}_2\text{-OCH}_2\text{CH}_2\text{N-cyclopropyl}$$

Compound	Substituent at X	Y	Z	log 1/C Obs.[a]	Calc.[b]	Δ(log 1/C)[c]
31	H	Br	H	6.64	6.40	0.24
32	Cl	Cl	H	6.30	6.46	-0.16
33	NO_2	H	H	5.76	5.68	0.08
34	CF_3	H	H	4.98	5.22	-0.24
35	H	CH_3	H	5.69	5.65	0.04
36	Cl	H	Cl	5.68	6.10	-0.42
37	Cl	CH_3	H	5.75	5.72	0.03
38	Br	H	H	5.64	5.95	-0.31
39	CH_3	Cl	H	6.06	5.47	0.59
40	Cl	H	H	5.82	6.04	-0.22
41	H	OCH_3	H	5.46	5.47	-0.01
42	CH_3	CH_3	H	4.71	4.73	-0.02
43	CH_3	H	CH_3	4.85	4.12	0.73
44	CH_3	H	H	4.78	5.05	-0.27
45	CH_3	Cl	CH_3	4.70	4.55	0.15
46	CH_3	CH_3	CH_3	3.54	3.81	-0.27
47	H	$N{=}NC_6H_5$	H	7.56	7.16	0.40
48	H	NH_2	H	4.40	4.74	-0.34

[a]Ref. 22. See footnote a, Table 4.8.

[b]Calculated using Equation 4.46.

[c]$(\log 1/C)_{obs} - \log (1/C)_{calc}$.

response. Table 4.11 summarizes the comparison between the observed and calculated response parameters.

In review, in the selection of series of compounds for subjection to the Hansch analysis, it is best to study many substituent changes in one position of the parent molecule before consideration of substitutional changes at multiple positions. In this way, one may be able to determine which substituent position is more critical to the activity of the compound if there is a difference. Careful consideration should then be given the series to determine if any of the congeners should be deleted from the analysis for apparent reasons. Certain compounds may be omitted from the analysis for any of several a priori reasons. Apparent steric restrictions (23-25), high chemical reactivity of a congener (23,26, 27), susceptibility to metabolic transformations (25), or the unavailability of reliable substituent parameters (28,29) may be good reasons.

After the preliminary analysis has been performed, other congeners might be omitted from further consideration due to large deviations from the equation describing most of the series (23,28,29). In addition, the proper choice of the biological response parameter is a prerequisite to the success of the analysis. Biological data should be accurate, quantitative, and measured under uniform conditions. Furthermore, the particular response parameters should be on an equiresponse or equidosage basis. That is, the data should represent the molar concentration of compound necessary to elicit a defined response or the response level resulting from a defined dosage.

Following the selection of a series of compounds and their resulting biological response data, one must then select an initial set of physicochemical parameters for inclusion in the LFER equation. Again, the basic physico chemical parameters include hydrophobic (Table 3.1), steric (Table 3.2), electronic (Table 3.3), or miscellaneous (Table 3.4). If one has an idea about the mechanism of action of the series, he is in a better position to choose parameters for trial correlations. Some investigators prefer to include parameters, when in doubt, and let the statistics provide further guidance in narrowing the number of parameters in the "final" equation. It is best, of course, that the particular parameter values selected should be those derived from systems as similar to the system to which they are to be applied as possible

REFERENCES

1. N. R. Draper and H. Smith, Applied Regression Analyses, John Wiley and Sons, Inc., New York, 1966.
2. J. D. P. Graham and M. A. Kamar, J. Med. Chem. 6, 103 (1963).
3. T. Fujita, J. Iwasa, and C. Hansch, J. Amer. Chem. Soc. 86, 5175 (1964).
4. A. Leo, C. Hansch, and D. Elkins, Chem. Revs. 71, 525 (1971).
5. P. Bracha and R. D. O'Brien, J. Econ. Entomol. 59, 1255 (1966).
6. C. Hansch and S. M. Anderson, J. Med. Chem. 10, 745 (1967).
7. C. Hansch, J. E. Quinlan, and G. L. Lawrence, J. Org. Chem. 33, 347 (1968).
8. J. Iwasa, T. Fujita, and C. Hansch, J. Med. Chem. 8, 150 (1965).
9. C. Hansch, A. R. Steward, S. M. Anderson, and D. Bentley, J. Med. Chem. 11, 1 (1968).
10. H. W. Smith, J. Phys. Chem. 25, 605 (1921).
11. H. W. Smith, J. Phys. Chem. 25, 204 (1921).
12. L. P. Hammett, Physical Organic Chemistry, McGraw-Hill, New York, 1940.
13. J. E. Leffler and E. Grunwald, Rates and Equilibria of Organic Reactions, John Wiley and Sons, Inc., New York, 1963.
14. D. H. McDaniel and H. C. Brown, J. Org. Chem. 23, 420 (1958).
15. P. R. Wells, Linear Free Energy Relationships, Academic Press, New York, 1968.
16. R. W. Taft in Steric Effects in Organic Chemistry, M. S. Newman, Ed., p. 556, John Wiley and Sons, Inc., New York, 1956.
17. M. Charton, J. Org. Chem. 29, 1222 (1964).
18. C. Hansch and E. J. Lien, Biochem. Pharmacol. 17, 709 (1968).
19. H. H. Jaffé, Chem. Rev. 53, 191 (1953).
20. A. Cammarata, R. C. Allen, J. K. Seydel, and E. Wempe, J. Pharm. Sci. 59, 1496 (1970).
21. E. Kutter and C. Hansch, J. Med. Chem. 12, 647 (1969).
22. R. W. Fuller, M. M. Marsh, and J. Mills, J. Med. Chem. 11, 397 (1968).
23. C. Hansch and E. W. Deutsch, Biochim. Biophys. Acta 112, 381 (1966).
24. C. Hansch, E. W. Deutsch, and R. N. Smith, J. Amer. Chem. Soc. 87, 2738 (1965).

25. C. Hansch, R. M. Muir, T. Fujita, P. P. Maloney, F. Geiger, and M. Streich, J. Amer. Chem. Soc. 85, 2817 (1963).
26. C. Hansch and E. W. Deutsch, Biochim. Biophys. Acta 126, 117 (1966).
27. C. Hansch and A. R. Steward, J. Med. Chem. 7, 691 (1964).
28. E. Miller and C. Hansch, J. Pharm. Sci. 56, 92 (196
29. W. P. Purcell, J. A. Singer, K. Sundaram, and G. L. Parks, "Quantitative Structure-Activity Relationshi and Molecular Orbitals in Medicinal Chemistry," in Medicinal Chemistry, 3rd ed., Chapter 10, A. Burger Ed., John Wiley and Sons, Inc., New York, 1970.

CHAPTER V

DE NOVO MODEL: THEORY AND DESCRIPTION

The principal objective in drug research is to uncover that one compound which is the most efficient for the treatment of a given disease or condition. The rational approach to this very complicated problem is (a) to measure the effectiveness of a wide variety of likely candidates (i.e., broad spectrum screening) in order to determine the class or classes of compounds which offer the greatest potential and (b) to seek the most active analog in the most active class.

The QSAR technique is of no help in the first step which involves finding a "lead compound." It does, however, represent perhaps the best hope for systematically minimizing the expense, delay, and work required for the second step.

In essence, the QSAR approach is an attempt to obtain maximum utilization and understanding from the activity data collected for a relatively small series of congeneric molecules in order to understand better the nature of the observed activity and to predict which untested analogs are the most likely candidates for synthesis.

If one wishes to apply the LFER model for a particular series of compounds, one must obtain, in addition to the biological response, values for the various physicochemical properties of these molecules which might dictate the magnitude of the activity. There is nothing to guarantee that, once one has gone to the trouble of calculating and/or measuring these parameters, a significant level of correlation of activity with any one or combination of these will be found.

The Free-Wilson model sometimes presents an opportunity to circumvent this problem. The price paid for this convenience is that, usually, more analogs must be studied initially, the results of an analysis using this model reveal less about the mode of action, and activity predictions cannot be made for a compound containing a substituent which was not included as an observation in the original analysis.

Suppose one has a series of congeneric molecules, each of which may be thought to consist of a "parent" compound (portion of the structure common to every molecule in the series), and two or more substituents (which vary from one member of the series to the next). The basic assumption of the Free-Wilson model is that, insofar as variations in activity from one molecule in the series to the next are concerned, activity of a given molecule can be expressed as the sum of contributions of the particular substituents on that molecule plus a constant. Thus, for a molecule with substituents A and B (e.g., $-CH_3$ and -Cl) and corresponding substituent contributions to activity S(A), S(B), the observed activity is assumed expressable as

$$\text{activity} = S(A) + S(B) + \mu \quad (5.1)$$

where μ is a constant. The immediate object is to obtain numerical values for the substituent contributions.

Suppose one has activity data, e.g., LD_{50}, "METD," etc., for the four hypothetical molecules represented by

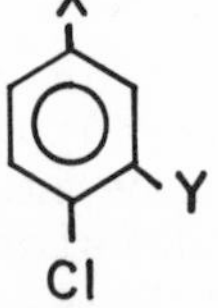

X

Y

Cl

$X = A_1, A_2$

$Y = B_1, B_2$

The chloro-benzene portion corresponds to the "parent" while the substituents A_1 and A_2 occur at position (segment) X and substituents B_1 and B_2 at position (segment) Y. The biological activity, β, for each analog can be expressed as

$$\beta_1 = S(A_1) + S(B_1) + \mu \quad (5.2)$$

$$\beta_2 = S(A_1) + S(B_2) + \mu \quad (5.3)$$

$$\beta_3 = S(A_2) + S(B_1) + \mu \tag{5.4}$$

$$\beta_4 = S(A_2) + S(B_2) + \mu \tag{5.5}$$

where $S(A_1)$ is the substituent contribution to the activity for substituent A_1, etc., and μ is the average of the observed β; μ is sometimes referred to as the contribution of the "parent" or unsubstituted part of the molecule. Free and Wilson further specify that the substituents at each segment (X and Y) must obey a "symmetry equation" which requires that the net contribution, summed over all biological activity equations as 5.2-5.5 above, of the substituents at each segment is zero; i.e., in this example,

$$2S(A_1) + 2S(A_2) = 0 \tag{5.6}$$

$$2S(B_1) + 2S(B_2) = 0 \tag{5.7}$$

Although these symmetry requirements appear to be, and are in one respect, somewhat arbitrary, they furnish constraints needed if unique solutions for the substituent contributions are to be obtained.

For the simple example now being discussed, Equations 5.2-5.7 can be solved to obtain values for the substituent contributions, $S(A_1)$, etc., in terms of the biological activities $\beta_1, \ldots \beta_4$. For such a solution one must assume that the biological phenomenon is perfectly described by this additivity model and that the observed biological data have been determined with no experimental error. In reality, neither of these can be expected to be true. In practice, the model will provide only an approximation (sometimes very crude) while the experimental data might contain errors of the magnitude of the activity index itself. Accordingly, one's only recourse is to take a statistical approach. This requires that each substituent at a given segment be represented a number of times (at the very least, twice) in the series of molecules in order that its activity contribution be assessed with some assurance of its appropriateness.

The same statistical measures of goodness of fit can be used in application of the Free-Wilson model as were discussed in Chapter II for the LFER models, namely, R^2, F (overall), EV, and the t-test for individual coefficient (substituent contribution) significance. Because of the large number of adjustable parameters, R^2 is not as sensitive a measure of fit as it is for the LFER models. The t values for the individual substituent contributions are usually very revealing and often, within a single analysis, point to confidence levels varying from <75% to >99%.

This is often a direct reflection of the number of times a particular substituent appears in the series of molecules considered.

Once a Free-Wilson analysis has been carried out an the mentioned statistical quantities calculated, one fir assesses the goodness of fit of the Free-Wilson model to the biological problem at hand. A high level of correla tion (e.g., R^2, EV $\geq$ 0.90; F (overall) ---> > 90% confidence level) implies that the assumptions inherent in th model can considered reasonable approximations. As one would expect, the statistics for a given problem will also depend on the accuracy and precision of the experimental biological data.

If it is decided that the Free-Wilson model can indeed "explain" the experimental findings, then the substituent contributions can be used to predict biological activities for analogs which have not been tested. For example, for a hypothetical series, such as

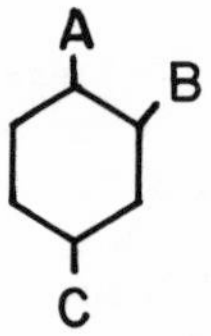

$A = A_1, A_2, A_3$

$B = B_1, B_2, B_3$

$C = C_1, C_2, C_3$

II

there are 3 X 3 X 3 = 27 possible analogs. Let the mole cule with A_1 at A, B_1 at B, and C_1 at C be represented a (A_1, B_1, C_1), etc. One does not need experimental biolo gical data on all 27 analogs in order to carry out a Fre Wilson analysis. Indeed, there would be no point in carrying out the analysis if <u>all</u> the answers are known. From the total set, one can select a number of subsets, so long as each substituent occurs in the subset at leas twice. For example, one might choose to evaluate experimentally the seven particular molecules represented as (A_1, B_1, C_1), (A_1, B_1, C_2), (A_2, B_2, C_1), (A_2, B_2, C_2), (A_3, B_3, C_3), (A_3, B_3, C_1), (A_1, B_2, C_3). If the observe activities of these molecules are $\beta_1, \beta_2, \ldots \beta_7$ respectively, then the corresponding set of Free-Wilson equations (including the symmetry equations), will be

$$S(A_1) + S(B_1) + S(C_1) + \mu = \beta_1 \tag{5.8}$$

$$S(A_1) + S(B_1) + S(C_2) + \mu = \beta_2 \tag{5.9}$$

$$S(A_2) + S(B_2) + S(C_1) + \mu = \beta_3 \qquad (5.10)$$

$$S(A_2) + S(B_2) + S(C_2) + \mu = \beta_4 \qquad (5.11)$$

$$S(A_3) + S(B_3) + S(C_3) + \mu = \beta_5 \qquad (5.12)$$

$$S(A_3) + S(B_3) + S(C_1) + \mu = \beta_6 \qquad (5.13)$$

$$S(A_1) + S(B_2) + S(C_3) + \mu = \beta_7 \qquad (5.14)$$

$$3S(A_1) + 2S(A_2) + 2S(A_3) = 0 \qquad (5.15)$$

$$2S(B_1) + 3S(B_2) + 2S(B_3) = 0 \qquad (5.16)$$

$$3S(C_1) + 2S(C_2) + 2S(C_3) = 0 \qquad (5.17)$$

where $S(A_1)$ is the substituent contribution for substituent A_1, etc., and $\mu = \Sigma_{i=1}^{7}\beta_i/7$. One can solve this system of linear equations to obtain numerical values for $S(A_1)$, $S(A_2)$ . . .$S(C_3)$. Using these quantities, one can then predict activities for the remaining twenty analogs. For example, the activity for the untested molecule (A_2, B_3, C_1) would be obtained as

$$\beta = S(A_2) + S(B_3) + S(C_1) + \mu \text{ etc.} \qquad (5.18)$$

The greater the number of locations at which substituents vary, and the greater the number of substituents considered at each location (segment), the greater the savings this technique potentially provides.

The Free-Wilson model can be used most effectively if the requirements for its successful application are taken into consideration when it is being decided which analogs are to be tested. In the preceeding example it is possible to select subsets containing up to 15 molecules and still not be able to apply this method. In particular, the compounds form such a series.

$(A_1B_1C_1)$	$(A_2B_2C_3)$	$(A_2B_3C_2)$
$(A_1B_1C_2)$	$(A_3B_3C_1)$	$(A_2B_3C_3)$
$(A_1B_1C_3)$	$(A_3B_3C_2)$	$(A_3B_2C_1)$
$(A_2B_2C_1)$	$(A_3B_3C_3)$	$(A_3B_2C_2)$
$(A_2B_2C_2)$	$(A_2B_3C_1)$	$(A_3B_2C_3)$

One might note that no individual substituent occurs less than three times in the series which contains nine unknown substituent contributions to be obtained (along with the regression constant) from fifteen experimental activity equations (along with three symmetry equations). Despite having (a) each substituent present in more than one compound and (b) more equations than unknowns, the system is nonetheless, unsolvable. The problem here is that two of the substituents, A_1 and B_1, occur only on the same molecules. That is, whenever A_1 is present, B_1 is also present on the same molecule. Therefore, no information (experimental activity) is available which can possibly allow one to separate the contribution of A_1 from that of B_1. Algebraically, the problem is that one does not have as many <u>independent</u> equations as unknowns.

Chapter VI

DE NOVO MODEL: PROCEDURE AND EXAMPLES

Since the introduction of the additive mathematical model by Free and Wilson in 1964, very few applications of the model have appeared in the literature. In their original paper Free and Wilson analyzed the biological activities of ten tetracycline antibiotics and the analgetic activities of 29 indanamines and were able to account for 91% and 81% of the variance of the data of the two series, respectively (1). In 1965, Purcell used this model in the correlation of the butyrylcholinesterase inhibitory potencies of twelve alkyl substituted 3-carbamoylpiperidines with their molecular structure. On the basis of these calculations, he predicted the activities of 26 other congeners (2). Four years later, in 1969, these predictions proved to be quantitative when one of these "predicted" derivatives was actually synthesized and tested biochemically (3). The calculated I_{50} value (molarity of the compound effecting 50% inhibition) of 1-decyl-3-(N-ethyl-N-methylcarbamoyl)piperidine hydrobromide was reported to be 0.78×10^{-5}M. Three years later, the experimental I_{50} value of this compound was found to be $0.98 \times 10^{-5} \pm 0.003 \times 10^{-5}$M, which is in good agreement with the predicted value. This was the first reported successful prediction of the biological activity of a compound by use of the *de novo* model (3).

Smithfield and Purcell have applied this model to the study of the hypoglycemic activities of twelve piperidinesulfamylsemicarbazides. From this analysis, they were able to predict the activities of twelve more analogs. The correlations between the calculated and observed biological responses agreed quantitatively (4). In another study, Purcell and Clayton have used the mathematical model in attempting to correlate the antitumor activities of numerous acetylemic carbamate derivatives (5). Although the statistics of the correlation are misleading due to the inclusion of several equations with substituent groups observed only once (resulting in a necessary "perfect" calculated biological activity for that equation), a good fit by the model was obtained upon the deletion of these groups in the analysis.

More recently (1969, 1971) Ban and Fujita have used the mathematical model of Free and Wilson in two separat structure-activity studies (6,7). In an initial analysi of the norepinephrine-uptake inhibition potencies of a number of sympathomimetic amines, they demonstrated that the biological responses of the series could be analyzed by the constant and additive activity contributions of the substituents and the parent phenethylamine skeleton (6). Using the square of the correlation coefficient (r^2) as a measure of the explained variance, they were able to account for 85% and 96% of the variance in the data using the standard response parameter and its logarithm, respectively, as suggested by Purcell and Clayton (5). Their quantitative correlation led Ban and Fujita to suggest that the conformation of the parent skeleton at the receptor site would not be changed markedly even if substituents are introduced into it. From their calculations the inhibitory activities of several untested compounds were predicted (6).

The second study by Fujita and Ban involved application of the Free-Wilson technique to several phenethylamine derivatives as substrates of enzymes associated wit the biosynthetic pathway of sympathetic transmitters (7) Obtaining quantitative structure-activity correlations, they found that the logarithmic activity data were usefu in analyzing the activities of the series in terms of th sum of contributions of structural fragments to free energy change in the enzyme-substrate complex formation (7).

In one recent additional application of this model, Hudson, Bass, and Purcell have studied the correlation between selected chloroquine derivatives and their minimum effective therapeutic dose against *Plasmodium gallinaceum* (8). They were able to obtain a correlation with a level of significance at the 95% confidence level (F-test) while explaining 78% of the variance. They als presented the basis for the statistical analysis of the model, the statistical tests involved in interpretation of the results, and some of the problems of ill conditioning in the analysis (8).

As is readily seen, when compared to other methods of quantitative structure-activity analyses, there are relatively few literature examples of the application of the mathematical (Free-Wilson) model.

METHODOLOGY

Of course, the utility of the quantitative structure-activity models lies in the ability to apply the method to one's own series of compounds of interest. The desired goal of such an analysis is to be able (1) to rank the substituent group activities noting possible structure-activity relationships such as the substituent position most critical to the activity of the compound and (2) to predict those compounds of the series not tested and possibly not synthesized which would have the greatest potential as biologically active compounds. In order to hope to realize these goals, several general prerequisites in addition to the basic concepts outlined in the previous chapter should be followed in subjecting data to such an analysis. Most important is the need to exercise due thought in the selection of biological data to be treated. One should have a "feel" for the activity data before using it; that is, in addition to understanding the basic type of data he is using (e.g., type of test, units, etc.), one should be fully aware of its quantitative nature, its reproducibility and reliability to give an accurate measure of the potency of the compound, and its limitations. Of course, the biological activity data selected should be accurate while quantitative and should be measured under uniform conditions for the series of molecules studied. QSAR analyses can only hope to achieve the quantitative and reliability level of the data that is treated.

In addition to satisfying the requirements for the selection of biological response data, one must exercise equal thought and care in choosing the molecules in the series to be treated (5). Congeners in the series should be closely similar to increase the probability of a constant mechanism of action for the series. One should keep in mind the basic underlying concept of the method that the substituent group activity contributions to the selected response parameters must be intrinsically additive. It is also desirable to have a maximum number of degrees of freedom and, therefore, to have a high ratio of the number of observations to the number of unknown terms in the linear equation. This allows for a greater statistical significance in the analysis. Thus, care must be taken in the selection of which congeners in the series to include in the analysis and which to exclude. Preliminary analysis of the data using the Free-Wilson method may aid in the selection of which molecules, if any, should be deleted from the analysis in order to help to insure that all groups treated do indeed follow the intrinsic additivity prerequisite. As may be seen in the examples that follow, an analysis in which one or two substituent groups consistently lead to a large deviation between the calculated and observed response for a particular molecule may suggest the non additive nature of the group. Subsequent analyses in which these possible non additive groups have not been included which lead to better overall correlation of the data may help to suggest further their non additive nature. Further precaution should be made in the selection of data to avoid the potential problems resulting in ill-conditioned matrices. The treatment of the problem of ill-conditioning in the previous chapter should be reviewed to avoid this problem.

Once the series of molecules and their biological activities that are to be treated have been selected, the data should be prepared for the analysis. First, one should be cautious in the selection of the numbers to be used from the available response data. Numbers selected should be on an equiresponse (i.e., the dosage necessary to elicit a defined response) or response per defined dosage basis. Raw or random response numbers lead to meaningless analyses. If the data available are not on an equiresponse or equidosage level, the data should be adjusted to obtain this effect. For example, if the data were given as percentage inhibition of a defined tumor system per defined dose of compound per kg of test animal where varying dosages have been administered over the series of compounds as a result of toxicity studies on the compounds, the response values might be divided by the size of the dosage. This would result in obtaining modified equidosage data or percentage tumor inhibition per mg of drug per kg of test animal. Such treatment helps to obtain usable data for analysis which might seem to be untreatable.

The same hypothetical example treated in Chapter IV can be used nicely here to illustrate the stepwise procedure for applying the Free-Wilson model. Assume that biological activities are available for the 18 derivatives given in Table 6.1.

Table 6.1 Hypothetical Example: Free-Wilson Model

X				Y				Z				
H	F	Cl	Br	H	NO_2	CN	$COCH_3$	H	CH_3	C_2H_5	OCH_3	Log(1/C)
X				X				X				3.095
X				X					X			2.763
X					X					X		4.556
X					X						X	5.405
	X					X		X				5.921
	X					X			X			5.625
	X						X			X		4.931
	X						X				X	5.701
		X		X				X				3.852
		X		X					X			3.460
		X			X					X		5.332
		X			X						X	6.132
			X			X		X				5.701
			X			X			X			5.409
			X				X			X		4.690
			X				X				X	5.631
X						X					X	4.793
			X		X			X				5.121

Step 1. Following Equation (5.1), one may write Equations 6.1-6.18:

$$3.095 = [H]_x + [H]_y + [H]_z + \mu \tag{6.1}$$

$$2.763 = [H]_x + [H]_y + [CH_3]_z + \mu \tag{6.2}$$

$$4.556 = [H]_x + [NO_2]_y + [C_2H_5]_z + \mu \tag{6.3}$$

$$5.405 = [H]_x + [NO_2]_y + [OCH_3]_z + \mu \tag{6.4}$$

$$5.921 = [F]_x + [CN]_y + [H]_z + \mu \tag{6.5}$$

$$5.625 = [F]_x + [CN]_y + [CH_3]_z + \mu \tag{6.6}$$

$$4.931 = [F]_x + [COCH_3]_y + [C_2H_5]_z + \mu \tag{6.7}$$

$$5.701 = [F]_x + [COCH_3]_y + [OCH_3]_z + \mu \tag{6.8}$$

$$3.852 = [Cl]_x + [H]_y + [H]_z + \mu \tag{6.9}$$

$$3.460 = [Cl]_x + [H]_y + [CH_3]_z + \mu \tag{6.10}$$

$$5.332 = [Cl]_x + [NO_2]_y + [C_2H_5]_z + \mu \quad (6.11)$$

$$6.132 = [Cl]_x + [NO_2]_y + [OCH_3]_z + \mu \quad (6.12)$$

$$5.701 = [Br]_x + [CN]_y + [H]_z + \mu \quad (6.13)$$

$$5.409 = [Br]_x + [CN]_y + [CH_3]_z + \mu \quad (6.14)$$

$$4.690 = [Br]_x + [COCH_3]_y + [C_2H_5]_z + \mu \quad (6.15)$$

$$5.631 = [Br]_x + [COCH_3]_y + [OCH_3]_z + \mu \quad (6.16)$$

$$4.793 = [H]_x + [CN]_y + [OCH_3]_z + \mu \quad (6.17)$$

$$5.121 = [Cl]_x + [NO_2]_y + [H]_z + \mu \quad (6.18)$$

These resulting 18 equations contain 13 unknowns. In addition, however, the restriction (Chapter V, p. 91) that the summation of the group activity contributions at each substituent position must sum to zero must be applied:

$$0 = 5[H]_x + 4[F]_x + 5[Cl]_x + 4[Br]_x \quad (6.19)$$

$$0 = 4[H]_y = 5[NO_2]_y + 5[CN]_y + 4[COCH_3]_y \quad (6.20)$$

$$0 = 5[H]_z + 4[CH_3]_z + 4[C_2H_5]_z + 5[OCH_3]_z \quad (6.21)$$

Since these equations do not represent actual biological observations and real activity data, they must be incorporated into the 18 equations representing the pharmacological data. This prevents the possible trap of misleading statistical significance of the results. In order to incorporate these restrictions into the equations (6.1-6.18) describing the data, a "dependent variable" is selected in each of the symmetry equations (6.19-6.21) and it is solved in terms of the other independent variables. If $[H]_x$, $[COCH_3]_y$, and $[CH_3]_z$ are selected as the "dependent variable" in Equations 6.19, 6.20, and 6.21, respectively, these equations become Equations 6.22, 6.23, and 6.24:

$$[H]_x = -0.8[F]_x - [Cl]_x - 0.08[Br]_x \quad (6.22)$$

$$[COCH_3]_y = -[H]_y - 1.25[NO_2]_y - 1.25[CN]_y \quad (6.23)$$

$$[CH_3]_z = -1.25[H]_z - [C_2H_5]_z - 1.25[OCH_3]_z \quad (6.24)$$

These equations are then substituted for $[H]_x$, $[COCH_3]_y$, and $[CH_3]_z$ where they appear in Equations 6.1-6.18. Thus, Equations 6.1-6.18 become 6.25-6.42, respectively:

$$3.095 = -0.8[F]_x - [Cl]_x - 0.8[Br]_x + [H]_y + [H]_z + \mu \quad (6.25)$$

$$2.763 = -0.8[F]_x - [Cl]_x - 0.8[Br]_x + [H]_y - 1.25[H]_z - [C_2H_5]_z - 1.25[OCH_3]_z + \mu \quad (6.26)$$

$$4.556 = -0.8[F]_x - [Cl]_x - 0.8[Br]_x + [NO_2]_y + [C_2H_5]_z + \mu \quad (6.27)$$

$$5.405 = -0.8[F]_x - [Cl]_x - 0.8[Br]_x + [NO_2]_y + [OCH_3]_z + \mu \quad (6.28)$$

$$5.921 = [F]_x + [CN]_y + [H]_z + \mu \quad (6.29)$$

$$5.625 = [F]_x + [CN]_y - 1.25[H]_z - [C_2H_5]_z - 1.25[OCH_3]_z + \mu \quad (6.30)$$

$$4.931 = [F]_x - [H]_y - 1.25[NO_2]_y - 1.25[CN]_y + [C_2H_5]_z + \mu \quad (6.31)$$

$$5.701 = [F]_x - [H]_y - 1.25[NO_2]_y - 1.25[CN]_y + [OCH_3]_z + \mu \quad (6.32)$$

$$3.852 = [Cl]_x + [H]_y + [H]_z + \mu \quad (6.33)$$

$$3.460 = [Cl]_x + [H]_y - 1.25[H]_z - [C_2H_5]_z - 1.25[OCH_3]_z + \mu \quad (6.34)$$

$$5.332 = [Cl_x] + [NO_2]_y + [C_2H_5]_z + \mu \quad (6.35)$$

$$6.132 = [Cl]_x + [NO_2]_y + [OCH_3]_z + \mu \quad (6.36)$$

$$5.701 = [Br]_x + [CN]_y + [H]_z + \mu \quad (6.37)$$

$$5.409 = [Br]_x + [CN]_y - 1.25[H]_z - [C_2H_5]_z - 1.25[OCH_3]_z + \mu \quad (6.38)$$

$$4.690 = [Br]_x - [H]_y - 1.25[NO_2]_y - 1.25[CN]_y + [C_2H_5]_z + \mu \quad (6.39)$$

$$5.631 = [Br]_x - [H]_y - 1.25[NO_2]_y - 1.25[CN]_y + [OCH_3]_z + \mu \quad (6.40)$$

$$4.793 = -0.8[F]_x - [Cl]_x - 0.8[Br]_x + [CN]_y + [OCH3]_z + \mu \quad (6.41)$$

$$5.121 = [Cl]_x + [NO_2]_y + [H]_z + \mu \quad (6.42)$$

This gives a final set of 18 equations with only 10 unknowns. These equations are then converted to matrices (6.43, 6.44, 6.45) ready for solution:

$$\begin{bmatrix} -0.8 & -1.0 & -0.8 & 1.0 & 0.0 & 0.0 & 1.0 & 0.0 & 0.0 \\ -0.8 & -1.0 & -0.8 & 1.0 & 0.0 & 0.0 & -1.25 & -1.0 & -1.25 \\ -0.8 & -1.0 & -0.8 & 0.0 & 1.0 & 0.0 & 0.0 & 1.0 & 0.0 \\ -0.8 & -1.0 & -0.8 & 0.0 & 1.0 & 0.0 & 0.0 & 0.0 & 1.0 \\ 1.0 & 0.0 & 0.0 & 0.0 & 0.0 & 1.0 & 1.0 & 0.0 & 0.0 \\ 1.0 & 0.0 & 0.0 & 0.0 & 0.0 & 1.0 & -1.25 & -1.0 & -1.25 \\ 1.0 & 0.0 & 0.0 & -1.0 & -1.25 & -1.25 & 0.0 & 1.0 & 0.0 \\ 1.0 & 0.0 & 0.0 & -1.0 & -1.25 & -1.25 & 0.0 & 0.0 & 1.0 \\ 0.0 & 1.0 & 0.0 & 1.0 & 0.0 & 0.0 & 1.0 & 0.0 & 0.0 \\ 0.0 & 1.0 & 0.0 & 1.0 & 0.0 & 0.0 & -1.25 & -1.0 & -1.25 \\ 0.0 & 1.0 & 0.0 & 0.0 & 1.0 & 0.0 & 0.0 & 1.0 & 0.0 \\ 0.0 & 1.0 & 0.0 & 0.0 & 1.0 & 0.0 & 0.0 & 0.0 & 1.0 \\ 0.0 & 0.0 & 1.0 & 0.0 & 0.0 & 1.0 & 1.0 & 0.0 & 0.0 \\ 0.0 & 0.0 & 1.0 & 0.0 & 0.0 & 1.0 & -1.25 & -1.0 & -1.25 \\ 0.0 & 0.0 & 1.0 & -1.0 & -1.25 & -1.25 & 0.0 & 1.0 & 0.0 \\ 0.0 & 0.0 & 1.0 & -1.0 & -1.25 & -1.25 & 0.0 & 0.0 & 1.0 \\ -0.8 & -1.0 & -0.8 & 0.0 & 0.0 & 1.0 & 0.0 & 0.0 & 1.0 \\ 0.0 & 1.0 & 0.0 & 0.0 & 1.0 & 0.0 & 1.0 & 0.0 & 0.0 \end{bmatrix} \quad (6.43)$$

$$\begin{bmatrix} [F]_x \\ [Cl]_x \\ [Br]_x \\ [H]_y \\ [NO_2]_y \\ [CN]_y \\ [H]_z \\ [C_2H_5]_z \\ [OCH_3]_z \end{bmatrix} \quad (6.44)$$

$$\begin{bmatrix} 3.095 \\ 2.763 \\ 4.556 \\ 5.405 \\ 5.921 \\ 5.625 \\ 4.931 \\ 5.701 \\ 3.852 \\ 3.460 \\ 5.332 \end{bmatrix}$$

$$\begin{bmatrix} 6.132 \\ 5.701 \\ 5.409 \\ 4.690 \\ 5.631 \\ 4.793 \\ 5.121 \end{bmatrix} \qquad (6.45)$$

Step 2. The determination of the contributions of each group to the activity becomes, as in the LFER example, one of finding the best set of coefficients using the method of least squares. The methodology used in this solution is essentially the same as that used in the LFER model. Matrices to be solved are essentially the same. Initially the cross product matrix (the coefficients of the normal equations) is calculated and inverted followed by solution of the independent variables (i.e., the substituent activity contributions). However unlike the LFER model in the *de novo* model, each substituent group represents an independent variable thus greatly increasing the size of the matrices. Because of the complexity of these matrices, the detailed mathematics will not be presented here.

Solution of these equations either by hand or using a computer program such as that in Appendix III generates the coefficients or substituent group activity contributions listed in Table 6.2.

Step 3. From the solutions in Step 2, one can generate Table 6.2 which gives the activity contributions for each group. Clearly, one then has a ranking of these contributions and, therefore, is in a position to make predictions.

Step 4. Before any activity predictions should be attempted, one should first consider the statistical significance of the correlation. Using the same basic statistical tests as those used to evaluate the significance of the LFER model and as outlined in Chapter II, one is better able to determine the significance of the correlation. Similar to the LFER model, the calculated values of biological activity must first be obtained for comparison with the experimental values. This is accomplished by substituting the group activity parameters listed in Table 6.2 into Equations 6.1-6.18. For example, the calculated value of compound 1, Table 6.1, would be obtained by solving Equation 6.1. This procedure is given in Equation 6.46:

Table 6.2 Calculated Parent (μ) and Substituent Group Activity Contributions

Substituent Group	Activity Contribution
$[H]_x$	-1.121
$[F]_x$	1.032
$[Cl]_x$	-0.382
$[Br]_x$	0.846
$[H]_y$	-0.435
$[NO_2]_y$	0.860
$[CN]_y$	0.246
$[COCH_3]_y$	-0.948
$[H]_z$	-0.253
$[CH_3]_z$	-0.581
$[C_2H_5]_z$	-0.068
$[OCH_3]_z$	0.772
μ	4.895

$$(-1.121) + (-0.435) + (-0.253) + 4.895 = 3.086 \qquad (6.46)$$

Repeating this procedure for the remainder of the compounds yields Table 6.3.

From these values in Table 6.3, one is then able to calculate R^2, R, F, and E.V.

Multiple Correlation Coefficient, R, R^2 (Chapter II, Equation 2.14)

$$R^2 = \frac{\Sigma(\hat{Y}-\overline{Y})^2 =}{\Sigma(Y-\overline{Y})^2 =} \frac{(17.273)}{(17.283)} = 0.9994 \qquad (6.47)$$

Table 6.3 Comparison of Calculated and Observed Activities

	X				Y					Z			log 1/C		
Cpd.	H	F	Cl	Br	H	NO_2	CN	$COCH_3$	H	CH_3	C_2H_5	OCH_3	obs	calc[a]	Δ log 1/C[b]
1	1				1				1				3.095	3.086	0.009
2	1				1					1			2.763	2.759	0.004
3	1					1					1		4.556	4.566	-0.010
4	1					1						1	5.405	5.407	-0.002
5		1					1		1				5.921	5.921	0.0
6		1					1			1			5.625	5.593	0.032
7		1						1			1		4.931	4.912	0.019
8		1						1				1	5.701	5.752	-0.051
9			1		1				1				3.852	3.826	0.026
10			1		1					1			3.460	3.498	-0.038
11			1			1					1		5.332	5.306	0.026
12			1			1						1	6.132	6.146	-0.014
13				1			1		1				5.701	5.735	-0.035
14				1			1			1			5.409	5.407	0.002
15				1				1			1		4.690	4.725	-0.035
16				1				1				1	5.631	5.565	0.066
17	1						1					1	4.793	4.793	0.0
18			1			1			1				5.121	5.121	0.0
P-1		1					1					1		6.945	
P-2		1				1						1		7.559	
P-3				1			1					1		6.759	
P-4				1		1						1		7.373	

[a]Calculated from values in Table 6.2.

[b]$(\log 1/C)_{obs} - (\log 1/C)_{calc}$.

$$R = \sqrt{R^2} = \sqrt{0.9994} = 0.9996 \quad (6.48)$$

Significance of the Regression, F (Chapter II, Equation 2.15)

$$F = \frac{\Sigma(\hat{Y}-\overline{Y})^2/(k)}{\Sigma(Y-\hat{Y})^2/(n-k-1)} = \frac{(17.273)/(9)}{(0.013)/(16-9-1)} = 1181.06 \quad (6.49)$$

$F_{[9,8]} = 11.8$ at the 0.001 confidence level

Explained Variance, E.V. (Chapter II, Equation 2.16)

$$E.V. = 1 - \frac{\Sigma(\hat{Y}-Y)^2/(n-k)}{\Sigma(Y-\overline{Y})^2/(n-1)} = 1 - \frac{(0.013)/(18-9)}{(17.273)/(18-1)}$$

$$= 0.9982 \quad (6.50)$$

From these calculations it is apparent that the analysis was statistically significant at approximately the 99% level.

Step 5. If this were a "real" example, the following molecules might be suggested as having the greatest probability of high activity and, therefore, perhaps worthy of synthesis and evaluation. Using the activity contribution values listed in Table 6.2 one might note that the substituent groups contributing the most relative activity to the overall response values of the congeners include $[F]_X$, $[Br]_X$, $[NO_2]_Y$, $[CN_Y]$ and $[OCH_3]_Z$. Thus, molecules containing these substituent groups are suggested by the analysis as being the most promising molecules in the series for further testing, or possibly synthesis. The most promising predicted compounds would be compounds P-1 to P-4 in Table 6.3, none of which were included in the prior evaluation and possibly not synthesis. In addition, all four of these compounds exhibit significantly higher predicted activities than any of the congeners actually evaluated. The analysis also suggests that substituent positions X and Y appear to be the more important positions of the molecule in terms of eliciting biological response.

This treatment may be followed more easily by use of an actual example. The first example was taken from the original paper by Free and Wilson (1) and has been reanalyzed for this study. The data treated was originally reported by Spencer and co-workers in which they determine

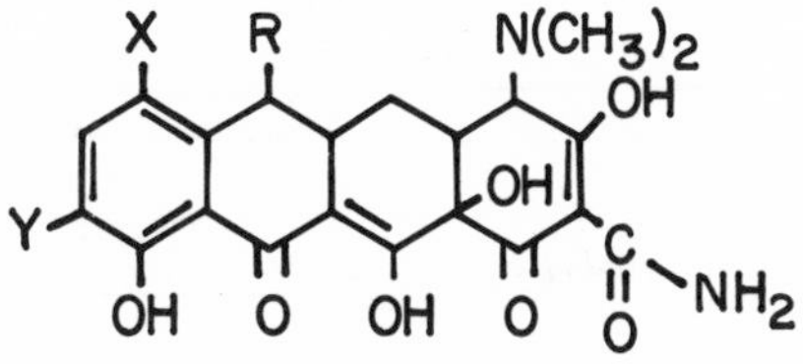

Compound Number	Substituents
I	R = H, X = Y = NO_2
II	R = H, X = Cl, Y = NO_2
III	R = H, X = Br, Y = NO_2
IV	R = H, X = Cl, Y = NH_2
V	R = H, X = Br, Y = NH_2
VI	R = H, X = NO_2, Y = NH_2
VII	R = CH_3, X = NO_2, Y = NH_2
VIII	R = CH_3, X = NO_2, Y = CH_3CONH
IX	R = CH_3, X = Br, Y = NH_2
X	R = CH_3, X = Br, Y = CH_3CONH

Figure 1

---

the *in vitro* inhibitory potencies of ten tetracycline derivatives against *Staphylococcus aureus* (Fig. 1) (9). The response parameters of compounds I-X were determined turbidimetrically relative to the standard of tetracycline with a biological activity of 100. These response parameters are given in Table 6.4. It should be noted that in this series a high biological response parameter is desirable.

Following the precautions and prerequisites outlined, one might consider the data quantitative, accurate, and measured under uniform conditions. Also, the data are of the response per equidosage type; therefore, it is

Table 6.4 *In Vitro* Inhibitory Potencies Against *Staphylococcus aureus* of Selected 6-Deoxytetracycline

Derivative of 6-deoxytetracycline	Biological Activity[a]
I, 6-demethyl-7,9-dinitro	60
II, 7-chloro-t-demethyl-6-nitro	21
III, 7-chloro-6-demethyl-9-nitro	21
IV, 9-amino-7-chloro-6-demethyl	525
V, 9-amino-7-bromo-6-demethyl	320
VI, 9-amino-6-demethyl-7-nitro	275
VII, 9-amino-7-nitro	160
VIII, 9-acetamido-7-nitro	15
IX, 9-amino-7-bromo	140
X, 9-acetamido-7-bromo	75

[a]Antibacterial activities measured by the turbidimetric assay using *Staphylococcus aureus* as the tested organism. Potencies are related to that of tetracycline having a value of 100 (9).

ready to be subjected to the analysis.

In the treatment of data by the quantitative structure-activity methods, the data should initially be set up in matrix form by substituent groups. The resulting matrix for the present series is shown in Table 6.5. In this table, the numeral 1 is placed under the column heading of the substituent group at each position in the compound. From this table then and by assuming the activity contributions of the substituent groups on the parent structure to be constant and additive to the total activity of the molecule, one can generate a linear equation for each observation of the general form of Equation 6.51:

$$\text{Biological Activity} = [R] + [X] + [Y] + \mu \qquad (6.51)$$

Table 6.5 Biological Activities of Selected Derivatives of 6-Deoxytetracycline Substituents at Position

	R			X			Y		
Compound	H	CH_3	NO_2	Cl	Br	NO_2	NH_2	CH_3CONH	Biological Activity[a]
I	1		1			1			60
II	1			1		1			21
III	1				1	1			15
IV	1			1			1		525
V	1				1		1		320
VI	1		1				1		275
VII		1	1				1		160
VIII		1	1					1	15
IX		1			1		1		140
X		1			1			1	75

[a]Footnote a, Table 6.4.

In 6.51, [R], [X], and [Y] represent the activity contribution to the total activity of a group substituted at positions R, X, and Y on the parent structure, respectively, while μ represents the overall average on the intrinsic activity of the parent moiety. The resulting equations for this series of compounds I-X are Equations 6.52-6.61, respectively:

$$[H]_R + [NO_2]_X + [NO_2]_Y + \mu = 60 \quad (6.52)$$

$$[H]_R + [Cl]_X + [NO_2]_Y + \mu = 60 \quad (6.53)$$

$$[H]_R + [Br]_X + [NO_2]_Y + \mu = 15 \quad (6.54)$$

$$[H]_R + [Cl]_X + [NH_2]_Y + \mu = 525 \quad (6.55)$$

$$[H]_R + [Br]_X + [NH_2]_Y + \mu = 320 \quad (6.56)$$

$$[H]_R + [NO_2]_X + [NH_2]_Y + \mu = 275 \quad (6.57)$$

$$[CH_3]_R + [NO_2]_X + [NH_2]_Y + \mu = 160 \quad (6.58)$$

$$[CH_3]_R + [NO_2]_X + [CH_3CONH]_Y + \mu = 15 \quad (6.59)$$

$$[CH_3]_R + [Br]_X + [NH_2]_Y + \mu = 140 \quad (6.60)$$

$$[CH_3]_R + [Br]_X + [CH_3CONH]_Y + \mu = 75 \quad (6.61)$$

In Equation 6.52, $[H]_R$ represents the activity contribution of a hydrogen moiety substituted at position R on the parent structure, $[NO_2]_X$ represents the activity contribution of the nitro group substituted at position X, and $[NO_2]_Y$ is the activity contribution of a nitro group at Y. μ is the activity contribution of the parent structure and 60 is the biological response parameter. Similarly, this follows for Equations 6.53-6.61. The total representation for the series results in ten equations with nine unknowns. In addition, the basic restrictions (or symmetry equations) that the sum of the group activity contributions at each substituent position must equal zero, according to the basic concepts of the method, were applied. This means, of course, that one equation is added to the set for each substituent position treated. In this example, one has three substituent positions, R, X, and Y, which lead to the addition of Equation 6.62, 6.63, and 6.64 for the substituent positions, respectively to the set:

$$6[H]_R + 4[CH_3]_R = 0 \qquad (6.62)$$

$$4[NO_2]_X + 2[Cl]_X + 4[Br]_X = 0 \qquad (6.63)$$

$$3[NO_2]_Y + 5[NH_2]_Y + 2[CH_3CONH]_Y = 0 \qquad (6.64)$$

These equations may not be entered directly into a regression analysis for the solution of the unknowns since they are not entirely independent. The regression analysis involved the simultaneous solution of linear independent equations. In addition, the direct inclusion of these equations would lead to misleading statistics concerning the analysis since indeed they do not represent additional independent observations and biological testing. These equations are generally incorporated into the analysis by selecting one of the variables in each equation and solving for it in terms of the other variables. Thus, with the resulting exclusion of one dependent variable for each substituent position in the solution of the equations, the number of unknowns to be solved is reduced by the number of substituent positions. Following this example, if one selects the activity contribution of CH_3 moiety as the dependent variable at substituent position R, Equation 6.65 results:

$$[CH_3]_R = -1.5[H]_R \qquad (6.65)$$

Similarly, if we select the substituent activity of the Cl moiety as the dependent variable at position X and the activity of the CH_3CONH- group as the dependent variable at position Y, we obtain Equations 6.66 and 6.67, respectively:

$$[Cl]_X = -2[NO_2]_X - 2[Br]_X \qquad (6.66)$$

$$[CH_3CONH]_Y = -1.5[NO_2]_Y - 2.5[NH_2]_Y \qquad (6.67)$$

Although any of the substituents at each position could have been selected as the dependent variable, these groups were selected since they represented the groups with the fewest observations. This results in some simplification of the data preparation.

The next step is the incorporation of the symmetry restrictions into the matrix (Table 6.5) set up for the series. Subsequent incorporation of these restrictions gives the resulting matrix shown in Table 6.6 and the Equations 6.68-6.77:

Table 6.6 Matrix Resulting from the Inclusion of Symmetry Restrictions and the Selection of $[CH_3]_R$, $[Cl]_X$, and $[CH_3CONH]_Y$ as Dependent Variables

	Substituents at Position					
	R	X		Y		
Compound	H	NO_2	Br	NO_2	NH_2	Biological Activity[a]
I	1	1		1		60
II	1	-2	-2	1		21
III	1		1	1		15
IV	1	-2	-2		1	525
V	1		1		1	320
VI	1	1			1	275
VII	-1.5	1			1	160
VIII	-1.5	1		-1.5	-2.5	15
IX	-1.5		1		1	140
X	-1.5		1	-1.5	-2.5	75

[a]Footnote a, Table 6.4

$$[H]_R + [NO_2]_X + [NO_2]_Y + \mu = 60 \tag{6.68}$$

$$[H]_R - 2[NO_2]_X - 2[Br]_X + [NO_2]_Y + \mu = 21 \tag{6.69}$$

$$[H]_R + [Br]_X + [NO_2]_Y + \mu = 15 \tag{6.70}$$

$$[H]_R - 2[NO_2]_X - 2[Br]_X + [NH_2]_Y + \mu = 525 \tag{6.71}$$

$$[H]_R + [Br]_X + [NH_2]_Y + \mu = 320 \tag{6.72}$$

$$[H]_R + [NO_2]_X + [NH_2]_Y + \mu = 275 \tag{6.73}$$

$$-1.5[H]_R + [NO_2]_X + [NH_2]_Y + \mu = 160 \tag{6.74}$$

$$-1.5[H]_R + [NO_2]_X - 1.5[NO_2]_Y - 2.5[NH_2]_Y + \mu = 15 \quad (6.75)$$

$$-1.5[H]_R + [Br]_X + [NH_2]_Y + \mu = 140 \quad (6.76)$$

$$-1.5[H]_R + [Br]_X - 1.5[NO_2]_Y - 2.5[NH_2] + \mu = 75 \quad (6.77)$$

These ten equations and the resulting six unknowns are then ready for simultaneous solution by the method of least squares either by hand or by means of a computer. A typical computer program for such a solution is given in Appendix II.

Lease-squares solution of the linear equations yields the calculated activity contribution of each substituent group as well as that of the parent structure. The substituent group contributions to the total activity are given for this example in Table 6.7. To obtain the

Table 6.7 Group Contributions to the Total Inhibitory Activities of Ten 6-Deoxytetracycline Derivatives

Substituent Position	Substituent	Activity Contribution[a]
R	H	75
R	CH_3	-113
X	Cl	84
X	Br	-16
X	NO_2	-26
Y	NH_2	123
Y	CH_3CONH	18
Y	NO_2	-218
μ	Parent moiety	161

[a]Footnote a, Table 6.4.

group contributions of these groups not actually solved (the dependent variables $[CH_3]_R$, $[Cl]_X$, $[CH_3CONH]_Y$) in the analysis, one needs only to "plug" those values determined for the groups treated in Equations 6.65, 6.66, and 6.67. For example, the value of $[CH_3]_R$ is obtained in the solution of Equation 6.78:

$$[CH_3]_R + -1.5[H]_R = -1.5(75) = -112.5 \tag{6.78}$$

Similarly, the values of $[Cl]_X$ and $[CH_3CONH]_Y$ are obtained in Equations 6.79 and 6.80:

$$\begin{aligned} [Cl]_X &= -2[NO_2]_X -2[Br]_X = -2(-26) -2(-16) \\ &= 84 \end{aligned} \tag{6.79}$$

$$\begin{aligned} [CH_3CONH]_Y &= -1.5[NO_2]_Y -2.5[NH_2] = -1.5(-218)-2.5(123) \\ &= 185 \end{aligned} \tag{6.80}$$

These values are also listed in Table 6.7.

The calculated total activity of each molecule may then be found by summation of this group contributions and μ. For example, for compound I where R=H, X=NO_2, Y=NO_2, the calculated total activity may be found by using the calculated values from Table 6.7 in Equation 6.52. Solution of Equation 6.52 yields Equation 6.81 in which the calculated activity of compound I was determined to be -8:

$$\begin{aligned} [H]_R + [NO_2]_X + [NO_2]_Y + \mu &= (75) + (-26) + (-218) + (161 \\ &= -8 \end{aligned} \tag{6.81}$$

Similarly, the calculated activities of the remainder of the congeners in the series may be determined. These values are given in Table 6.8.

Before the results of the analysis are examined too closely for structure-activity correlations, one should first determine the significance of the regression by subjecting the results to several statistical tests (Chapter II). The basic tests which should be considered are the coefficient of multiple correlation, R, the square of the coefficient, R^2, the amount of explained variance, and the level of significance of the regression from the F-ratio. Treating the differences between the observed and calculated biological response parameters, we obtain an R value of 0.95 and an explained variance as determined from R^2 of 90%. The other measure of explained variance yielded a value of 79%. The F ratio for the series was 7.68 indicating a 95-97.5% level of significance. The

Table 6.8 Observed and Calculated Biological Response Parameters of Selected 6-Deoxytetracycline Derivatives

	Substituent Positions									
	R		X			Y			Biological Activity	
Cpd.	H	CH_3	NO_2	Cl	Br	NO_2	NH_2	CH_3CONH	Observed[a]	Calculated
I	1		1			1			60	-8
II	1			1		1			21	102
III	1				1	1			15	2
IV	1			1			1		525	444
V	1				1		1		320	343
VI	1		1				1		275	333
VII		1	1				1		160	145
VIII		1	1					1	15	40
IX		1			1		1		140	155
X		1			1			1	75	50
P-I	1				1			1		2.37
P-II	1			1				1		

[a]Footnote a, Table 6.4.

difference between the estimated and observed activity would be due to biological variation in the *in vitro* procedure and/or a nonadditive component in the series. Thus, the statistics indicate a quantitative or significant correlation of the data.

One of the major values of the method lies in the ability to use the results of a significant correlation to study possible structure-activity relationships. First, the substituent groups should be ranked according to their activities as was done in Table 6.7 for this example. From these data the most active types of substituent groups as well as the more active substituent positions may be noted. In this example, the substituent positions seem to contribute approximately the same relative amounts to the total activity while the parent moiety is the major contributor. In this small series, very few structure-activity relationships are apparent.

A second value of the method lies in its potential to allow one to expand the series of compounds actually tested. This may be accomplished by the prediction of the activities of several compounds of the series not tested, and possibly not synthesized, which would have the greatest potential as biologically active agents. By the same method that the calculated biological response parameters are determined, one may also predict the activities of compounds composed of these same substituents which were not observed. For example, one might predict the activity of the derivative of the series in which R=H, X=Br, and $Y=CH_3CONH_2$, compound P-I in Table 6.8, to be 237, an activity value higher than most of the observe values. A second predicted response parameter of 338 might be calculated for the congener in which R=H, X=Cl, $Y=NH_2$ (Compound P-II, Table 6.8). In this way, the serie of data that was treated might be expanded to suggest potential molecules for synthesis and evaluation.

A second example of the application of the Free-Wilson analysis was given by Smithfield and Purcell and has been modified for illustration here (4). Studying the hypoglycemic activities of some piperidinesulfamylsemicarbazides (Fig. 2) which were reported by McManus and Gerber (10), they analyzed the data according to the <u>de novo</u> model.

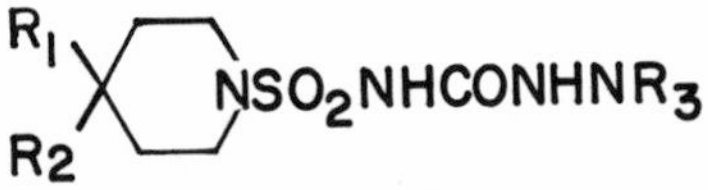

R_1, R_2 — $NSO_2NHCONHNR_3$

Figure 2

R_1 = H, CH_3, $(CH_2)_2$; R_2 = H, CH_3, $(CH_2)_2$, C_2H_5; R_3 = (CH$_2$
$(CH_2)_6$

In Fig. 2, the $(CH_2)_2$ substituent at position R_1 represents one half of a tetramethylene group $(CH_2)_4$ which is necessarily paired with the $(CH_2)_2$ at R_2. The data that were analyzed are given in Table 6.9 following the genera procedures outlined in the first example for setting up the matrix.

Table 6.9 Observed Hypogylcemic Activities of Ten Suhstituted Piperidinesulfamylsemicarbazides

Compound	Substituents at R_1				Substituents at R_2				Substituents at R_3		Biological Response[b]
	H	CH_3	C_2H_5	$(CH_2)_2$[a]	H	CH_3	C_2H_5	$(CH_2)_2$[a]	$(CH_2)_5$	$(CH_2)_6$	
I	1				1				1		14.8 ± 7.0
II	1				1					1	11.1 ± 1.9
III	1					1			1		26.1 ± 2.6
IV	1					1				1	33.9 ± 1.5
V		1				1			1		39.1 ± 2.8
VI		1				1				1	34.9 ± 3.3
VII		1					1			1	42.0 ± 3.3
VIII			1				1			1	34.4 ± 2.8
IX				1				1	1		35.6 ± 2.4
X				1				1		1	30.8 ± 3.7

[a]The 4,4-tetramethylene group is denoted by two units of $(CH_2)_2$, one each at positions R_1, and R_2.

[b]The activities are reported as maximum percent blood glucose lowering at a dose of 100 mg/kg with their standard deviations (10).

Those compounds in the series which contain substituent groups which were observed only once were deleted in this analysis since they result in necessarily perfect, quantitative fits in the analysis and yield misleading statistical tests. The biological parameters used in this study are the maximum percent fall in blood glucose per 100 mg of drug per kg of animal weight, a response per equidose parameter, reported by McManus and Gerber (10). The values listed in Table 6.9 include the standard deviations obtained in their experimental studies.

Following the procedure outlined in example 1, one may now generate one linear equation for each observation. These ten equations are given as Equations 6.82-6.91:

$$[H]R_1 + [H]R_2 + [(CH_2)_5]R_3 + \mu = 14.8 \quad (6.82)$$

$$[H]R_1 + [H]R_2 + [(CH_2)_6]R_3 + \mu = 11.1 \quad (6.83)$$

$$[H]R_1 + [CH_3]R_2 + [(CH_2)_5]R_3 + \mu = 26.1 \quad (6.84)$$

$$[H]R_1 + [CH_3]R_2 + [(CH_2)_6]R_3 + \mu = 33.9 \quad (6.85)$$

$$[CH_3]R_1 + [CH_3]R_2 + [(CH_2)_5]R_3 + \mu = 39.1 \quad (6.86)$$

$$[CH_3]R_1 + [CH_3]R_2 + [(CH_2)_6]R_3 + \mu = 34.9 \quad (6.87)$$

$$[CH_3]R_1 + [C_2H_5]R_2 + [(CH_2)_5]R_3 + \mu = 42.0 \quad (6.88)$$

$$[C_2H_5]R_1 + [C_2H_5]R_2 + [(CH_2)_6]R_3 + \mu = 34.4 \quad (6.89)$$

$$[(CH_2)_2]R_1 + [(CH_2)_2]R_2 + [(CH_2)_5]R_3 + \mu = 35.6 \quad (6.90)$$

$$[(CH_2)_2]R_1 + [(CH_2)_2]R_2 + [(CH_2)_6]R_3 + \mu = 30.8 \quad (6.91)$$

One might readily observe that there are more unknowns, 1 than there are equations or observations, ten of which leads to an insoluble situation. Even if there were as many as zero degrees of freedom (ten equations, ten variables), the situation would still lead to a statistically insignificant analysis, although soluble. However, after careful observation of the parent moiety, it appears to be a logical assumption that substituent positions might be considered equivalent. That is, the compound which contains a methyl (CH_3) group at position R_1 and a hydrogen (H) moiety at position R_2 would appear to be no different than the congener which has a H and CH_3 at position R_1 and R_2, respectively. By this assumption then, the variable $[H]R_1$ equals $[H]R_2$; $[CH_3]R_1$ is the same as

$[CH_3]R_2$; $[C_2H_5]R_1$ equals $[C_2H_5]R_2$; and $[(CH_2)_2]R_1$ equals $[(CH_2)_2]R_2$. This substitution then reduced the number of unknowns by 4 and thereby increases the number of degrees of freedom by 4. The resulting equations are given by Equations 6.92-6.101 and the new matrix is given in Table 6.10:

$$2[H]R_1,R_2 + [(CH_2)_5]R_3 + \mu = 14.8 \quad (6.92)$$

$$2[H]R_1,R_2 + [(CH_2)_6]R_3 + \mu = 11.1 \quad (6.93)$$

$$[H]R_1,R_2 + [CH_3]R_1,R_2 + [(CH_2)_5]R_3 + \mu = 26.1 \quad (6.94)$$

$$[H]R_1,R_2 + [CH_3]R_1,R_2 + [(CH_2)_6]R_3 + \mu = 33.9 \quad (6.95)$$

$$2[CH_3]R_1,R_2 + [(CH_2)_5]R_3 + \mu = 39.1 \quad (6.96)$$

$$2[CH_3]R_1,R_2 + [(CH_2)_6]R_3 + \mu = 34.9 \quad (6.97)$$

$$[CH_3]R_1,R_2 + [C_2H_5]R_1 + [(CH_2)_5] + \mu = 42.0 \quad (6.98)$$

$$2[C_2H_5]R_1,R_2 + [(CH_2)_6]R_3 + \mu = 34.4 \quad (6.99)$$

$$2[(CH_2)_2]R_1,R_2 + [(CH_2)_5]R_3 + \mu = 35.6 \quad (6.100)$$

$$2[(CH_2)_2]R_1,R_2 + [(CH_2)_6]R_3 + \mu = 30.8 \quad (6.101)$$

Symmetry equations for substituent positions R_1 (6.101) and R_3 (6.102) in which $[C_2H_5]R_1,R_2$ (6.104) and $[(CH_2)_5]R_3$ (6.105) are selected as the dependent variables are then incorporated into the matrix:

$$6[H]R_1,R_2 + 7[CH_3]R_1,R_2 + 3[C_2H_5]R_1,R_2 + 4[(CH_2)_2]R_1,R_2 = 0 \quad (6.102)$$

$$4[(CH_2)_5]R_3 + 6[(CH_2)_6]R_3 = 0 \quad (6.103)$$

$$[C_2H_5]R_1,R_2 = -2[H]R_1,R_2 - 2.33[CH_3]R_1,R_2 - 1.33[(CH_2)_2]R_1,R_2 \quad (6.104)$$

$$[(CH_2)_5]R_3 = -1.5[(CH_2)_6]R_3 \quad (6.105)$$

The resulting final matrix is given in Table 6.11. The ten equations with five unknowns represented in this matrix (6.106)-(6.115) are then solved simultaneously by the method of least squares:

$$2[H]R_1,R_2 - 1.5[(CH_2)_6]R_3 + \mu = 14.8 \quad (6.106)$$

Table 6.10 Reduced Matrix of the Observed Hypoglycemic Activities of Ten Substituted Piperidinesulfamylsemicarbazides

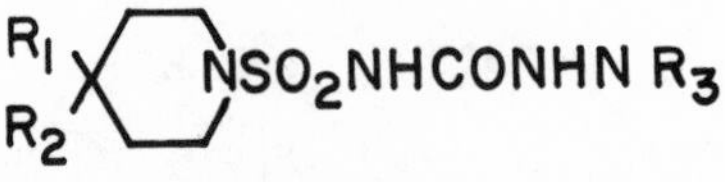

$R_1R_2C(CH_2CH_2)_2NSO_2NHCONHN R_3$

Compound	Substituents at R_1, R_2				Substituents at R_3		Biological Activity[b]
	H	CH_3	C_2H_5	$(CH_2)_2^{a}$	$(CH_2)_5$	$(CH_2)_6$	
I	2				1		14.8
II	2					1	11.1
III	1	1			1		26.1
IV	1	1				1	33.9
V		2			1		39.1
VI		2				1	34.9
VII		1	1			1	42.0
VIII			2			1	34.4
IX				2	1		35.6
X				2		1	30.8

[a]Footnote a, Table 6.9.

[b]Footnote b, Table 6.9.

Table 6.11 Final Matrix of the Observed Hypoglycemic Activities

Compound	Substituents at R_1, R_2			Substituent at R_3	Biological Activity[b]
	H	CH_3	$(CH_2)_2$[a]	$(CH_2)_6$	
I	2			-1.5	14.8
II	2			1	11.1
III	1	1		-1.5	26.1
IV	1	1		1	33.9
V		2		-1.5	39.1
VI		2		1	34.9
VII	-2	-1.33	-1.33	1	42.0
VIII	-4	-4.33	-2.66	1	34.4
IX			2	-1.5	35.6
X			2	1	30.8

[a]Footnote a, Table 6.11.
[b]Footnote b, Table 6.11.

$$2[H]R_1,R_2 + [(CH_2)_6]R_3 + \mu = 11.1 \quad (6.107)$$

$$[H]R_1,R_2 + [CH_3]R_1,R_2 - 1.5[(CH_2)_6]R_3 + \mu = 26.1 \quad (6.108)$$

$$[H]R_1,R_2 + [CH_3]R_1,R_2 + [(CH_2)_6]R_3 + \mu = 33.9 \quad (6.109)$$

$$2[CH_3]R_1,R_2 - 1.5[(CH_2)_6]R_3 + \mu = 39.1 \quad (6.110)$$

$$2[CH_3]R_1,R_2 + [(CH_2)_6]R_3 + \mu = 34.9 \quad (6.111)$$

$$-2[H]R_1,R_2 - 1.33[CH_3]R_1,R_2 - 1.33[(CH_2)_2]R_1,R_2 + [(CH_2)_6]R_3 + \mu = 42.0 \quad (6.112)$$

$$-4[H]R_1,R_2 - 4.33[CH_3]R_1,R_2 - 2.66[(CH_2)_2]R_1,R_2 + [(CH_2)_6]R_3 + \mu = 34.4 \qquad (6.113)$$

$$2[(CH_2)_2]R_1,R_2 - 1.5[(CH_2)_6]R_3 = 35.6 \qquad (6.114)$$

$$2[(CH_2)_2]R_1,R_2 - [(CH_2)_6]R_3 = 30.8 \qquad (6.115)$$

The resulting calculated substituent group constants including the values for $[C_2H_5]R_1,R_2$ and including the values for $[C_2H_5]R_1,R_2$ and $[(CH_2)_5]R_3$ calculated by Equation 6.104 and 6.105, respectively, and μ are given in Table 6.12. The groups are ranked according to their activity contributions at each substituent position.

Table 6.12 Calculated Substituent and Parent Group Activity Constants to Total Hypoglycemic Activities

Substituent Position	Group	Calculated Activity[a]
R_1,R_2	CH_3	4.36
R_1,R_2	C_2H_5	4.26
R_1,R_2	$(CH_2)_2$[b]	1.29
R_1,R_2	H	-8.07
R_3	$(CH_2)_5$	0.56
R_3	$(CH_2)_6$	-0.37
μ	Parent Structure	30.5

[a]Footnote b, Table 6.9.

[b]Footnote a, Table 6.9.

The calculated biological activities for the series were then calculated by the substitution of these values into Equations 6.91-6.100. These calculated values are given in Table 6.13. From the deviations between the observed and calculated biological responses, the statistical significance of the regression is determined. It is interesting to note that the calculated activities of

Table 6.13 Observed and Calculated Hypoglycemic Activities

	Substituents at R_1, R_2				Substituents at R_3		Biological Activity[a]		
Compound	H	CH_3	C_2H_5	$(CH_2)_2$[b]	$(CH_2)_5$	$(CH_2)_6$	obs[c]	calcd[d]	obs-calc
I	2				1		14.8 $\pm$ 7.0	14.90	-0.10
II	2					1	11.1 $\pm$ 1.9	13.97	-2.87
III	1	1			1		26.1 $\pm$ 2.6	27.33	-1.23
IV	1	1				1	33.9 $\pm$ 1.5	26.40	-7.50
V		2			1		39.1 $\pm$ 2.8	39.76	-0.66
VI		2				1	34.9 $\pm$ 3.3	38.83	-3.93
VII		1	1			1	42.0 $\pm$ 3.3	38.73	3.27
VIII			2			1	34.4 $\pm$ 2.8	36.47	-2.07
IX				2	1		35.6 $\pm$ 2.4	33.61	-1.99
X				2		1	30.8 $\pm$ 3.7	32.69	-1.89
P-I		1	1		1			39.68	
P-II			2			1		38.65	

[a]Activities are reported as the maximum percent lowering of blood glucose at a dose of 100 mg/kg (10).

[b]Footnote a, Table 6.9.

[c]Includes the standard deviation of the observed values.

[d]Calculated from Equations 6.87–6.96 using the values from Table 6.12.

only three of the ten compounds (Table 6.13, Compounds II IV, and VI) are outside the range of the experimental error of the observed values. The result of the statistical tests ($R = 0.94$, $R^2 = 0.89$, $F = 9.77$ for a level of significance of 97.5-99%, explained variance 80%) also indicate a relatively high level of significance for the regression analysis.

Using the results of the analysis to study possible structure-activity relationships, one might note that the parent structure does indeed contribute the majority of the activity to the compounds (as would be expected from most receptor theories). The activity contributions of the groups substituted in position R_1, R_2, however, appear to influence the overall activity of the compounds while the substituents studied in position R_3 have very little effect on this total activity. The activities of compounds in the series not reported may be predicted from these results (Table 6.13, Compound V). Although the compound with the greatest predicted activity from these results was included in the analysis, a compound (Table 6.13, Compound P-I) with CH_3 and C_2H_5 groups at R_1, R_2 and a $(CH_2)_5$ moiety at R_3 has approximately the same predicted activity. A second compound with C_2H_5 groups substituted at R_1, R_2 and a $(CH_2)_6$ moiety at R_3 (Table 6.13, Compound P-II) yields a predicted activity higher than most of those that were evaluated. Thus, the analyses again illustrate the utility of this method in suggesting potential compounds which might be worthy of synthesis and testing as possible therapeutic agents.

REFERENCES

1. S. M. Free, Jr., and J. W. Wilson, J. Med. Chem. 7, 395 (1964).
2. W. P. Purcell, Biochim. Biophys. Acta 105, 201 (1965).
3. J. G. Beasley and W. P. Purcell, Biochim. Biophys. Acta 178, 175 (1969).
4. W. R. Smithfield and W. P. Purcell, J. Pharm. Sci. 56, 577 (1967).
5. W. P. Purcell and J. M. Clayton, J. Med. Chem. 11, 199 (1968).
6. T. Ban and T. Fujita, J. Med. Chem. 12, 353 (1969).
7. T. Fujita and T. Ban, J. Med. Chem. 14, 148 (1971).
8. D. R. Hudson, G. E. Bass, and W. P. Purcell, J. Med. Chem. 13, 1184 (1970).
9. J. L. Spencer, J. J. Hlavka, J. Petisi, H. M. Krazinski, and J. H. Boothe, J. Med. Chem. 6, 405 (1963).
10. J. M. McManus and C. F. Gerber, J. Med. Chem. 9, 256 (1966).

APPENDIX I

EXPERIMENTAL DETERMINATION OF PARTITION COEFFICIENTS*

This Appendix describes methods for determining partition coefficients of organic compounds between 1-octanol and water. A general outline of procedure precedes discussion of three useful analytical techniques: ultraviolet and visible spectrophotometry, gas chromatography, and Nessler's analysis. In addition, there is a summary of several important conditions which should be observed during partitioning to minimize errors.

The octanol-water partition coefficient represents the distribution of a substance between an organic and aqueous phase. The ratio is defined as P = [C]octanol/ [C]H_2O. Since P is a quantity with no dimensions, any units of concentration are appropriate. P is not independent of concentration and, ideally, infinite dilutions should be used in the calculations. However, for neutral compounds which have little tendency to associate, 10^{-1} M is sufficiently dilute. For acids and other molecules which tend to associate, measurements should be made at several concentrations and log P plotted against concentrations to obtain the value at infinite dilution. For very lipophilic molecules, one must work below the critical micelle concentration in the aqueous phase. This may be as low as 10^{-5}M (1).

Partition coefficients of molecules which react with water to yield ions must be corrected for ionization and expressed as the partition coefficient of the neutral or

*The authors are indebted to Corwin Hansch for making this description, which is his own, available through personal communication.

ionized species. For example,

$$R_3N + H_2O \rightleftharpoons R_3NH^+ + OH^-$$

I II

Alternatively, one may run the partitioning at a pH where only one species is present. For this purpose 0.1N HCl or 0.1N NaOH may be used. Depending on the ionization constant of the amine, the degree of dilution, and whether the solution is buffered or not, one may have varying proportions of I and II. If the pH of the buffer is high enough, all of the amine may be kept in the form of I and no correction is necessary. If not, a correction must be made as follows:

$$P = \frac{[C]_{octanol}}{(1-\alpha)\,[C]_{H_2O}}$$

where α is the degree of ionization.

Partitioning. The general procedure is to dissolve a carefully weighed sample of compound completely in the phase in which it is most soluble. The calculated amount of the second phase is added, the bottles shaken (about two minutes, by hand). The bottles are then placed in a centrifuge and turned at about 2000 rpm for one to two hours. An aliquot of one phase is withdrawn and analyzed.

Compound Preparation. Care must be taken to see that compounds to be measured are quite pure. The purity of liquids can usually be checked by gas chromatography and solids by thin layer chromatography. Melting points and boiling points are not good standards of purity.

Weighing. Accurate weighing is quite important. A large enough sample should be used so that the percent error is considerably under 1%. If one is employing a balance accurate to 0.1 mg, a 20-mg sample might have an error of 0.5%. Care must be taken to see that no loss occurs in transferring the sample to the partitioning bottle. We have found that small microscope cover glasses are convenient so that cover glass and sample can be carefully dropped into the partitioning bottle, minimizing loss of solids. Liquids can be weighed in small glass tubes and the whole tube placed in the solvent.

Partition Bottles. Ideal bottles are handmade with ground-glass stoppers. It is convenient to partition an centrifuge in the same bottle. For general use, 250 ml capacity is a convenient size. Centrifuging is most important and incomplete separation of the two phases is one of the most serious sources of error. For many compounds rubber stoppers are satisfactory; however, some compounds are strongly absorbed by rubber and poor results may be obtained with these.

Solvents. Even the best grade of commercial octano contains impurities which may affect the analysis. Octa nol should be purified by washing it with 10% sodium hydroxide, dilute sulfuric acid and, finally, bicarbonat solution. After drying over magnesium sulfate, it is di tilled under reduced pressure (b.p. ∿80°/2 mm). Careful fractionation through an efficient column of the first 10% or so of material removes the impurities which absor in the untraviolet region so that the rest of the materi may be rapidly distilled. Small amounts of impurities d not affect partition coefficients although they may affe the analysis. Its purity should be checked by gas chrom tography. The octanol is then shaken with distilled wat to saturate it.

When pipeting octanol, much longer times are necess to properly drain pipets because octanol is more viscous than water. Ordinary distilled water is satisfactory fo most work except with Nessler's reagent, which requires water free of ammonia. The distilled water should be saturated with octanol. For neutral compounds, small changes in the pH of the aqueous phase have little effec however, for ionized compounds this is quite important (see below).

Dissolving Compounds for Partitioning. Often it is quite difficult to dissolve certain compounds in either phase. Finely powdering the solid compounds helps in their dissolution. Heating may be employed to aid the process, but care must be taken to see that on cooling a true solution is obtained and not a supersaturated solution. Adding a very tiny crystal is sufficient to induc crystallization if indeed a supersaturated solution has been obtained. Allowing the mixture to shake overnight will solve some solution problems.

Mixing. The phases are usually mixed by inverting the bottles at least 60 times by hand during approximate two minutes. Studies by Craig (1) indicate that when th phases are of about equal volume, equilibrium is rapidly attained. When high ratios (e.g., 2 ml octanol and 200 ml H_2O) are used, longer shaking is necessary. Care must be taken to avoid vigorous shaking or serious emulsification may result. Such emulsions can be broken by allowing long standing and longer centrifugation; putting such emulsions through millipore filters also aids in breaking them.

To minimize error in calculating, the phases should be adjusted in volume so that roughly equal weights of compounds end up in each phase. Sometimes one must deviate from this ideal situation with molecules with extremely low or high P values. It must be borne in mind that results will be less reliable when one divides very small numbers into large numbers.

Care must be taken so that after partitioning each phase is still undersaturated. One way of checking on this point is to determine partition coefficients using several different concentrations of substance. A constant value indicates that no special interaction of substrate is occurring in either phase and that neither phase is saturated.

Centrifugation. Routinely, the partitioned phases are centrifuged for two hours at 2000 rpm. Shorter or longer times are appropriate, depending on the emulsification propensity. If emulsification is detected after two hours spinning, allowing the mixture to stand overnight and recentrifugation the next day usually solves the problem. Continued appearance of emulsions may indicate that shaking is too violent. A visual comparison of partitioned sample with pure water helps in detecting small amounts of emulsifications. This must be completely removed for accurate work. Large errors can result, especially with highly lipophilic compounds if cloudiness is not completely removed.

With some highly surface active compounds it may be necessary to allow the phases to stand for several days instead of centrifuging.

Sampling. Ideally, samples of each phase should be analyzed and the partition coefficient calculated from the two separate values. In this way a material balance can be made to insure against unforseen losses. This is often inconvenient and time consuming since an analytical procedure must be worked out for each phase. Since partitioning must be done at more than one concentration to be sure that special interactions are not occurring and to check against other errors, a rather large effort is necessary for one P value. Reliable results can be obtained by analyzing only one phase, but running four separate partitionings at different concentrations. The amount of solute found in one phase is then substracted from the total sample to obtain the amount in the second phase. The four runs serve to insure against an unforseen loss as well as checking for dependence of P on dilution. Standard curves are always run in duplicate, using two separate weighings of solute to be sure that no errors have been made in this critical reference. With few exceptions, log P values are obtained with a standard deviation of 0.03 units or less. Compounds with log P outside the range of ± 3.0 are of course most difficult to run. However, by using compounds with stronger u.v. absorbance, it is possible to obtain log P values from -5 to +5. This allows one to place on a single reference scale (octanol and water) compounds whose partition coefficients vary by 10^{10}.

Most often it is the aqueous phase from which one wishes to take a sample. This can be done by thrusting a pipet with a finger over the top through the octanol phase into the aqueous phase. A small amount of air should be blown through to force out any octanol which may have entered the tip. A thin, long needle syringe is even better for such sampling.

Standards. A carefully weighed sample is dissolved, usually in water, and diluted in a volumetric flask to produce a standard solution. With some very insoluble molecules, dissolving them first in a few ml of methanol and then diluting greatly aids the solution process. If the methanol concentration does not exceed 5%, this does not change the absorbance. Methanol should also be employed in the blank.

A simpler alternative method is to dissolve a sample of the compound to be partitioned in octanol-saturated water. Its absorbance can be measured with the spectrophotometer or its peak area determined with gas chromatography. A portion of the water is then partitioned and the absorbance or peak area of the water layer determined. The difference in the two measurements gives the amount of material in the octanol phase after partitioning. This method suffers from a number of serious disadvantages: If the absorbance does not follow Lambert-Beer's law and the concentration in water before and after partitioning is large, a serious error could result without one's knowing it. The technique cannot be used if methanol is used to dissolve the sample. Unless the partition coefficient is relatively near 1, it is not convenient to make runs using reasonable ranges of concentrations; also, unless one weighs out the sample, concentrations in the phases are unknown. This technique is most useful with gas chromatography (see below).

Spectrophotometry. Spectrophotometry is, in general, the more convenient method of analysis. The method is, of course, limited to compounds having strong extinction coefficients. Some typical values for monosubstituted benzenes from the compilation of Dyer (2) are given in Table I.

Note that in the case of the OH group (function 7), it is more easily detected by converting it into its ionic form (function 14).

The absorbance spectrum of each compound is taken from about 350-400 mμ down to 240 mμ where octanol begins to absorb. Having the complete spectrum is quite useful because one can compare the spectra before and after partitioning. Sometimes changes are seen which may be due to small amounts of impurities which do not follow the compound being partitioned; this serves as an additional check on purity. This also serves to detect any shift in the zero point due to emulsion formation. The peak where strongest absorption occurs is used for analysis unless it occurs below 240 mμ. A blank of centrifuged water saturated with octanol is employed.

A stable zero point base line with both cuvettes containing octanol-saturated water or octanol-saturated buffer is first set. Dilutions of the standard should be run to confirm adherence to Beer's law in the concentration region where one expects to work.

When analyzing very dilute solutions or poor absorbers, a 10-centimeter cell can be helpful. Under these conditions octanol-saturated water is difficult to work with as a standard. For those compounds which absorb considerably above 240 mμ, a pure water blank may be used with little loss in accuracy.

When working with acids and bases, one should check carefully the wavelength at which maximum absorbance occurs. A shift in the point of absorbance may be due to too dilute buffer.

Calculation of the Partition Coefficient. Extinction coefficients should be the same from two different standards. If they are not the same, but close in value, they may be averaged. When Beer's law is not followed, then a

Table I C_6H_5-X

	X	Primary band λ max, mμ	ε max
1	H	203.5	7,400
2	NH_3^+	203.	7,500
3	CH_3	206.5	7,000
4	I	207.	7,000
5	Cl	209.5	7,400
6	Br	210.	7,900
7	OH	210.5	6,200
8	OCH_3	217.	6,400
9	SO_2NH_2	217.5	9,700
10	CN	224.	13,000
11	CO_2^-	224.	8,700
12	CO_2H	230.	11,600
13	NH_2	230.	8,600
14	O^-	235.	9,400
15	$NHCOCH_3$	238.	10,500
16	$COCH_3$	245.5	9,800
17	CHO	249.5	11,400
18	NO_2	268.5	7,800

graph must be made and concentration determined by extrapolation.

1. Invert extinction coefficient = C/A = (mg standard/ml) absorbance.

2. Multiply by absorbance of aliquot of partitioned phase to find concentration:

$$(C/A)_{standard} \times A_{partitioned\ phase} = C = mg/ml$$

3. Multiply volume of partitioned phase (usually H_2O):

mg/ml X ml in partitioned phase = mg in phase

4. Subtract weight in this phase from original sample weight:

sample wt. - wt. in H_2O = weight in octanol

5. Take ratio:

$$\frac{\text{mg in octanol/vol octanol}}{\text{mg } H_2O/\text{vol } H_2O} = P$$

Gas Chromatography. Compounds which do not absorb strongly enough for spectrophotometric analysis may be analyzed by gas chromatography. After some practice to develop sample techniques, good results can be obtained although, in general, accuracy is not so good as the spectrophotometric method. With few exceptions, log P values have been obtained with standard deviations from four samples of ± 0.05 or less using a Loenco Model 70 with hydrogen flame detector. A good general reference for theory as well as choice of columns, experimental conditions, and so on is McNair and Bonelli (3).

To separate the octanol and water peaks from the sample, the most generally useful columns are SE-30, carbowax 20M or Apiezon L columns. Optimum working conditions must be established before analysis and carefully maintained throughout the injection of the standard and partitioned samples. To attain maximum sensitivity, constant volumes are injected into the column at a given attenuation.

Often it is convenient and feasible to use the standard solution for partitioning. One to 10 μl aliquots of standard or partitioned phase are used. Injections are made until three to five peaks of essentially equal size are obtained. For best results, the partitioned peak of the standard (or one of its dilutions) should be of similar size to that of the partitioned phase.

The peaks are then cut out with scissors and weighed to find their relative area and the weights averaged.

Some workers prefer to Xerox the lightweight chart paper onto heavier paper before cutting it to obtain pieces easier to weigh. The difference in weight between the standard peak and the sample peak represents the amount of sample in the second phase.

$$P = \frac{\text{(wt. std. peak)(dilution)} - \text{(wt. partitioned peak)}}{\text{Wt. Partitioned peak}}$$

$$\times \frac{\text{vol } H_2O}{\text{vol. octanol}}$$

Nessler's Analysis. Amides, ureas, carbamates, and certain other compounds which yield ammonia may be analyzed by this technique. Many such compounds absorb poorly in the u.v. and are so polar that they are difficult to analyze by gas chromatography. In the Nessler method (4) which is quite sensitive, the nitrogen-containing compoun is hydrolyzed to free ammonia which is combined with mercuric iodide to yield a colored product:

$$ROC(=O)\text{-}NH_2 \xrightarrow{H_2O} NH_3$$

$$2K_2HgI_4 + 2NH_3 \rightarrow H_2NHg_2I_3 + 4KI + NH_4I$$

Since ammonia is a common contaminate of the laboratory atmosphere, extra care is needed to exclude it. Ordinary distilled water is not sufficiently free of ammonia and should be redistilled or deionized.

For compounds which are easily hydrolyzed, 25 ml of the partitioned aqueous phase is added to 100 ml of 10% sodium hydroxide in a 250-ml round-bottom flask. Tight-fitting connections must be used. The flask is fitted with a distilling head, condenser, and adaptor. The adaptor is immersed in 10 ml of standard 1% hydrochloric acid. About 20 ml of water is distilled into the flask containing the hydrochloric acid. The acid solution is then added to a 50-ml volumetric flask and diluted to volume. The receiver must of course be carefully rinsed and these washings also added to the volumetric flask. Standards and partitioned aliquots are all diluted to the same volume. Two standards with two distillations per standard are run to insure that complete hydrolysis has occurred. [With more stable amides, acid hydrolysis of a more vigorous nature must be carried out (4).] Between each run the entire apparatus must be rinsed with deionized water. The partitioned phase is also analyzed in duplicate.

Nessler's reagent should be prepared several days in advance. The procedure is:

1. Dissolve 100 g HgI_2 and 70 g Kl in approximately 75 ml H_2O.
2. Dissolve 160 g NaOH in about 700 ml H_2O.
3. Combine the two solutions and dilute to 1 liter. Allow the precipitate to settle and use the clear yellow supernatant. A blank should be run on the distilled water each day to insure that the reagent has not decomposed.

To a 25-ml aliquot, 1/2 ml of Nessler's reagent (use pipet) is added. Good stirring is necessary during the addition. A magnetic stirrer is handy for this operation. Exactly five minutes is allowed for color development and the absorbance is read at 410 mμ.

Conditions which influence the color development and must be held constant are: temperature, pH, time of mixing, and rate of addition of reagent. If a red precipitate occurs during analysis, the solution is too acidic; this can be corrected by adding several drops of 50% sodium hydroxide to the distillate before diluting and developing with Nessler's reagent.

Temperature Dependence. The partition coefficient is not very sensitive to changes in temperature (1,16) if the phases employed are quite immiscible in each other. In this sense, octanol-water makes a good reference system. Our own unpublished results indicate that in the temperature range 0-25°, log P varies about 0.005 to 0.01 units/degree. A small amount of published work supports these findings (5,6). Therefore, partitioning at room temperature without temperature control is sufficient for most purposes.

Intermolecular Interactions of Solute Molecules. Although not yet completely understood, a rather large variety of interactions of solute molecules may occur so that it is not easy to be sure exactly what the nature of the species undergoing partitioning is. The behavior of aliphatic acids can be quite complex. In addition to the dissociation:

$$RCOOH + H_2O \rightleftharpoons RCOO^- + H_3O^+$$

which can be controlled by proper buffering, dimerization can occur in two possible ways:

$$\text{RCOOH} \rightleftharpoons \text{R-C}\begin{matrix}\nearrow\!\!\!\!= \text{O}\cdots\text{HO}\searrow \\ \searrow \text{OH}\cdots\text{O}\!=\!\!\!\nearrow\end{matrix}\text{C-R}$$

$$2\text{HOOC} \sim\!\sim\!\sim\!\sim \rightarrow \text{HOOC} \approx\!\approx\!\approx \text{COOH}$$

The first of the above two ways of dimerization is not important in dilute aqueous solution; however, this reaction is favored in apolar solvents such as cyclohexane or benzene. In octanol it does not appear (7) to be very significant at or below 10^{-3}M. Dimerization by the entwinement of long aliphatic chains at concentrations below the critical micelle concentration is not well understood (8), but definite evidence for it exists (9). Constant values of partition coefficients for such compounds are difficult if not impossible to obtain. Micelle formation in the aqueous phase must also be avoided. Such an occurrence cannot necessarily be detected visually; one must work below the critical micelle concentration if it is known (10). If it is not known, P should be determined at more and more dilute concentrations until a constant value is reached; this will probably entail the use of radioactive molecules.

Volatile Compounds. To eliminate weighing errors, the standard solution can be directly added to the second phase. In such examples it is sometimes advantageous to use ratios of absorbance rather than standard curves. For very volatile compounds, a correction for the amount partitioned into area above the phases may be necessary (7). Glass-stoppered cuvettes minimize evaporation while running spectra. The air space in the partitioning bottle above the phases should be held to a minimum for volatile compounds by employing almost enough of the two phases to fill the flask.

Problems of Instability. Certain compounds hydrolyze slowly in aqueous solution or are oxidized by air. Such adverse reactions can be minimized by carrying out the work as rapidly as possible in a cold room (4°). The error due to temperature will, in some cases, be less than that due to the chemical changes at higher temperature. Several different standards should be run to check for significant changes in the solute.

Solvent Volumes. Since most organic compounds are more soluble in octanol than water, one normally uses less octanol than aqueous phase. In addition to improved accuracy, this conserves octanol and its recovery. Adjustment of solvent volumes can decrease analytical error. For example, for a compound having P = 200, if one employed equal volumes of 100-ml and a 20-mg sample,

$$P = \frac{20}{.1 \text{ mg}}$$

An error of $\pm$.05 mg in the aqueous phase means that P = 133 - 400

By adjusting the solvents to 200 ml H_2O and 5 ml of octanol, we find

$$P = \frac{17.5}{3.5} \times \frac{200}{5} = 200$$

Now an error of $\pm$.05 mg in the aqueous phase yields P = 197 - 203.

Standard Deviation. With molecules which absorb strongly in the u.v. whose log P values are between -2.0 and +2.0, a standard deviation for four samples of 0.01 log units can be obtained. For compounds having higher or lower log P values, wider standard deviations are found (see above).

$$S.D. = \sqrt{\frac{\Sigma (X_i - X)^2}{n-1}}$$

X_i = log P value
x = average log P value
n = number of determinatio[n]

Pyridine is a good compound for the beginner to check his technique. Using octanol and distilled water, one should find log P = 0.65$\pm$.01. A more rigorous test of technique can be made with toluene, which is more volatile. With this compound one should be able to obtain log P = 2.69 $\pm$.02.

Acids and Bases. When most investigators use the term partition coefficient, they are referring to the unionized form of the acids or bases. With amines, the difference between P for the protonated species ($R_3\overset{+}{N}H$) over the neutral species (R_3N) is usually about 3 to 4 powers of 10 or 3 to 4 log units in the octanol-water system. For acids, the difference between log P for

COOH and COO^- is 4 to 4 log units. Therefore, very little of the ionized species goes with the neutral form into the octanol phase; in fact, for practical purposes, it is assumed to be zero.

Compounds with dissociation constants less than 10^{-7} need not be buffered, and no correction is necessary. With such neutral molecules, distilled water may be employed as the aqueous phase. For stronger acids and bases, it is desirable to choose a buffer such that at least 50% of the solute is unionized. Low concentrations of inorganic salts ($\leq$1M) do not appear to affect partition coefficients; however, larger changes in pH may. Selection of proper pH becomes especially tricky with amphoteric compounds such as sulfa drugs and amino acids. For the latter is the pH of the isoelectric point is generally selected, assuming that this places the solute in the form

$$\begin{array}{c} RCHCOO^- \\ | \\ NH_3^+ \end{array}$$

For compounds having an acidic and basic group, an intermediate pH value of buffer can be selected so that one has mostly neutral molecules.

The apparent partition coefficient of an acid or base is

$$P = \frac{[C]\text{undissociated (octanol)}}{[C]\text{undissociated } (H_2O) + [C]\text{dissociated } H_2O}$$

To correct this value, one divides only by the fraction ionized (1-α), where α is the fraction of compound dissociated in the water phase. For further details see Albert and Serjeant (13). The value of α can be calculated as follows:

$$\text{(a) for acids, } \alpha = \frac{1}{1 + \text{antilog}(pK_a - pH)}$$

$$\text{(b) for bases, } \alpha = \frac{1}{1 + \text{antilog}(pH - pK_a)}$$

Using the values in Table II from Albert and Serjeant (13) one can illustrate the correction for N-acetylanthranilic acid.

Table II Calculations of Percentage Ionized, Given pK_a and pH

pK_a - pH	If Anion	If Cation
-6.0	99.99990	0.0000999
-5.0	99.99900	0.0009999
-4.0	99.9900	0.0099990
-3.5	99.968	0.0316
-3.4	99.960	0.0398
-3.3	99.950	0.0501
-3.2	99.937	0.0630
-3.1	99.921	0.0794
-3.0	99.90	0.09991
-2.9	99.87	0.1257
-2.8	99.84	0.1582
-2.7	99.80	0.1991
-2.6	99.75	0.2505
-2.5	99.68	0.3152
-2.4	99.60	0.3966
-2.3	99.50	0.4987
-2.2	99.37	0.6270
-2.1	99.21	0.7879
-2.0	99.01	0.990
-1.9	98.76	1.243
-1.8	98.44	1.560
-1.7	98.04	1.956
-1.6	97.55	2.450
-1.5	96.93	3.07
-1.4	96.17	3.83
-1.3	95.23	4.77
-1.2	94.07	5.93
-1.1	92.64	7.36
-1.0	90.91	9.09
-0.9	88.81	11.19
-0.8	86.30	13.70
-0.7	83.37	16.63
-0.6	79.93	20.07
-0.5	75.97	24.03
-0.4	71.53	28.47
-0.3	66.61	33.39
-0.2	61.32	38.68
-0.1	55.73	44.27
0	50.00	50.00

Table II Continued

pK_a - pH	If Anion	If Cation
+0.1	44.27	55.73
+0.2	38.68	61.32
+0.3	33.39	66.61
+0.4	28.47	71.53
+0.5	24.03	75.97
+0.6	20.07	79.93
+0.7	16.63	83.37
+0.8	13.70	86.30
+0.9	11.19	88.81
+1.0	9.09	90.91
+1.1	7.36	92.64
+1.2	5.93	94.07
+1.3	4.77	95.23
+1.4	3.83	96.17
+1.5	3.07	96.93
+1.6	2.450	97.55
+1.7	1.956	98.04
+1.8	1.560	98.44
+1.9	1.243	98.76
+2.0	0.990	99.01
+2.1	0.7879	99.21
+2.2	0.6270	99.37
+2.3	0.4987	99.50
+2.4	0.3966	99.60
+2.5	0.3152	99.68
+2.6	0.2505	99.75
+2.7	0.1991	99.80
+2.8	0.1582	99.84
+2.9	0.1257	99.87
+3.0	0.09991	99.90
+3.1	0.0794	99.921
+3.2	0.0630	99.937
+3.3	0.0501	99.950
+3.4	0.0398	99.960
+3.5	0.0316	99.968
+4.0	0.0099990	99.9900
+5.0	0.0009999	99.99900
+6.0	0.0000999	99.99990

$P_{observed}$ = 29.0
pK_a = 3.63
pH of buffer = 3.81
$P_{corrected} = \frac{29}{0.398} = 74$

pK_a - pH = -0.18
% ionized = 60.2*
= .602
1- = 0.398
log P = 1.86

*Value obtained by interpolation between.
From Albert and Serjeant (13). Used with permission.

Additive-Constitutive Character of Log P. Since one can make quite reasonable estimates (7,14,15,16) of log P using log P or π values for known similar molecules, it is best to do so before commencing the measurement of an unknown partition coefficient. In this way one can determine in advance the optimum values of each of the solvent phases to be used. The log P of a fraction of a molecule is defined as: $\pi_X = \log P_X - \log P_H$ where P_X is the partition coefficient of a derivative and P_H that of a parent compound. For example, π for the CH_3 group can be found as follows:

$$\pi_{CH_3} = \log P_{toluene} - \log P_{benzene}$$

The values of π have been determined for most common functions (7) using several different parent systems. Except where there is strong electronic or steric interaction between substituent (7), π is an additive function. Alkyl functions appear to be quite insensitive to electronic effects and each CH_3 or CH_2 unit has a π value of $0.50 \pm .02$ for both aliphatic and aromatic compounds. Otherwise, π values for aromatic substituents (15) are quite different from those of aliphatic functions.

Sample calculation for dodecyl alcohol:

$$\log P_{ethanol} + 10\pi_{CH_2} = \log P_{dodecyl\ alcohol}$$

$$\begin{aligned} \log P_{dodecyl\ alcohol} &= -0.16 + 10(.5) = 5.16 \\ &= \text{calcd value} \\ 5.13 &= \text{expt value} \end{aligned}$$

Branching in an alkyl chain lowers log P or π by about 0.02 and a double bond lowers these values by 0. 3 units. Example:

Expt log P for 2-butanol = 0.61

Calcd log P for butanol $= .34(\log P_{propanol}) + .50 = .84$

The π value for -CH=CHCH=CH- obtained as an average of 9 values from different systems is 1.35. Log P for pyridine is 0.65. Acridine can then be calculated as follows:

$$2\pi_{C_4H_4} + \log P_{pyridine} = 2.70 + 0.65 = 3.35$$

The experimentally found value is 3.40.

In certain instances there appears to be interaction between the π electrons of an aromatic ring and polar side chain functions which lowers partition coefficients. For example, log $P_{benzene}$ = 2.13. This value plus 3(.5) = calcd value of 3.63 for n-propyl benzene. The measured value is 3.69; however, log $P_{benzene}$- log $P_{propanol}$ = 2.13 + 3.4 = 2.47. The experimental value (14) for $C_6H_5CH_2CH_2CH_2OH$ = 1.88. The difference of 0.6 appears to be due to interaction of the OH with the benzene ring. Such a possibility for interaction is not present in the hydrocarbon benzene. Log P for diethylstilbestrol may be calculated as follows:

$$\text{Hexane} - \pi_{\text{double bond}} - \pi_{\text{2 branchings}} + 2 \log P_{\text{phenol}}$$

$$= 3.00 - 0.30 - 2(0.2) + 2(1.46) = 5.22 \text{ calc}$$

$$5.07 \text{ obsd}$$

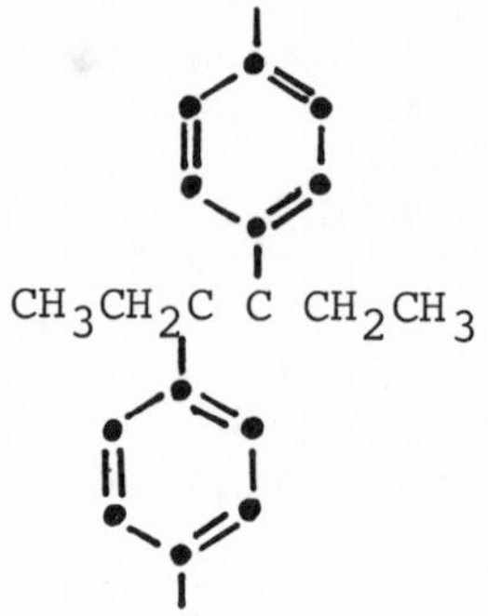

CH_3CH_2C C CH_2CH_3 diethylstilbestrol

REFERENCES

1. L. C. Craig and D. Craig in Technique of Organic Chemistry, Vol. III, p. 1, Chapter 4, Interscience Publishers, New York, 1950.
2. J. C. Dyer, Applications of Absorption Spectroscopy of Organic Compounds, p. 18, Prentice-Hall, Englewood Cliffs, N.J., 1965.
3. H. M. McNair and E. J. Bonelli, Basic Gas Chromatography, Varian, 2700 Mitchell Drive, Walnut Creek, California. 94598 (1965).
4. D. F. Boltz, Ed., Chemical Analysis, Vol. VIII, p. 84, Interscience Publishers, New York, 1958.
5. I. Wark, Proc. Roy. Soc. N.S. Wales 63, 47 (1929).
6. G. S. Forbes and A. S. Coolidge, J. Am. Chem. Soc. 41, 150 (1919).
7. T. Fujita, J. Iwasa and C. Hansch, J. Am. Chem. Soc. 86, 5175 (1964).
8. J. L. Kavanu, Structure and Function in Biological Membranes, Vol. I, Chapter 2, Holden Day Inc., San Francisco, California, 1965.
9. P. Mukerjee and K. J. Mysels, J. Phys. Chem. 62, 1390, 1400 (1958).
10. K. B. Klevens, J. Am. Oil Chem. Soc. 30, 74 (1953).
11. W. Scholtan, Arzneim. Forsch. 18, 505 (1968).
12. T. Koizumi, T. Arita, and K. Kakemi, Chem. Pharm. Bull. 12, 413 (1964).
13. A. Albert and E. P. Serjeant, Ionization Constants of Acids and Bases, Methuen and Co. Ltd., London, 1962.
14. J. Iwasa, T. Fujita, and C. Hansch, J. Med. Chem. 8, 150 (1965).
15. C. Hansch and S. M. Anderson, J. Org. Chem. 32, 2583 (1967).
16. A. Leo, C. Hansch, and D. Elkins, Chem. Rev. 71, 525 (1971).

APPENDIX II

MATRIX SOLUTION OF LFER EXAMPLE IN CHAPTER 4.

Initially, matrices of the forms II.1-II.3 are generated for the series of equations:

$$\begin{bmatrix} y_1 \\ y_2 \\ y_3 \\ \cdot \\ \cdot \\ \cdot \\ y_n \end{bmatrix} \tag{II.1}$$

$$\begin{bmatrix} x_{11} & x_{12} & \cdots & x_{1k} \\ x_{21} & x_{22} & \cdots & x_{2k} \\ \cdot & & & \\ \cdot & & & \\ \cdot & & & \\ x_{n1} & x_{n2} & \cdots & x_{nk} \end{bmatrix} \tag{II.2}$$

$$\begin{bmatrix} b_1 \\ b_2 \\ b_3 \\ \cdot \\ \cdot \\ \cdot \\ b_k \end{bmatrix} \quad \text{(II.3)}$$

In the first matrix (II.1) y represents the biological response parameters, log 1/C, for compounds 1 through n where n is the total number of equations or observations, 8 in this example, yielding an 8 X 1 matrix (II.4).

$$\begin{bmatrix} 3.095 \\ 6.000 \\ 5.201 \\ 5.631 \\ 3.425 \\ 5.420 \\ 5.401 \\ 5.290 \end{bmatrix} \quad \text{(II.4)}$$

In the second matrix (II.2) $x_{11}, x_{12}, \ldots x_{1k}$ represent the independent variables or physicochemical parameters being treated in the analysis from 1 through k where k is the total number of types of parameters being treated. In this example, only two independent variables or physicochemical parameters, π and σ, are being considered; therefore, k = 2 and $x_{11}, x_{21}, \ldots x_{81}$ represent the $\Sigma\pi$ values and $x_{12}, x_{22}, \ldots x_{82}$ are the $\Sigma\sigma$ parameters. This results in the 8 X 2 matrix (II.5):

$$\begin{bmatrix} \underline{\pi} & \underline{\sigma} \\ 0.000 & 0.000 \\ 0.370 & 1.115 \\ 1.410 & 0.963 \\ 0.690 & 1.008 \\ 0.120 & 0.115 \\ 1.340 & 1.045 \\ 0.950 & 0.964 \\ 0.570 & 0.893 \end{bmatrix} \quad \text{(II.5)}$$

Matrix II.3 represents the partial regression coefficient or the coefficients of the independent variables π and σ. Thus b_1 represents a and b_2 represents b in equation 4.1. This 2 X 1 matrix is given in Equation II.6.

$$\begin{bmatrix} a \\ b \end{bmatrix} \tag{II.6}$$

The value of c (Equation 4.1) is then determined from the calculated values of a and b.

The actual mechanical solution of the equations involves the solution of other matrices determined from the elements of these three matrices rather than by their direct solution. The actual matrix equation to be solved is given in Equation II.7,

$$\underset{\underline{A}}{\begin{bmatrix} a_{11} & a_{12} & \cdots & a_{1k} \\ a_{21} & a_{22} & \cdots & a \\ \vdots & & & \\ a_{k1} & a_{k2} & \cdots & a_{kk} \end{bmatrix}} \underset{\underline{B}}{\begin{bmatrix} b_1 \\ b_2 \\ \vdots \\ b_k \end{bmatrix}} = \underset{\underline{C}}{\begin{bmatrix} c_1 \\ c_2 \\ \vdots \\ c_k \end{bmatrix}} \tag{II.7}$$

in which $\underline{A}$ is a matrix of the coefficients of the normal equations whose elements are determined by Equation II.8 and $\underline{C}$ represents the constant terms of these normal equations calculated from Equation II.9:

$$a_{hj} = a_{jh} = n \sum_{i=1}^{n} x_{hi} X_{ji} - \sum_{i=1}^{n} x_{hi} \Sigma x_{ji} \tag{II.8}$$
$$(h = 1, 2, \ldots k; \quad j = 1, \ldots k)$$

$$c_h = n \sum_{i=1}^{n} x_{hi} Y_i - \sum_{i=1}^{n} x_{hi} \sum_{i=1}^{n} y_i \tag{II.9}$$
$$(h = 1, 2, \ldots K)$$

Substituting π and σ values into these equations for our example results in the 2 X 2 matrix (II.10) for values of a_{hj} determined from Equations II.11-II.13:

$$\begin{bmatrix} 15.42 & 9.16 \\ 9.16 & 10.95 \end{bmatrix} = 84.94 \qquad \text{(II.10)}$$

$$a_{11} = 8 \sum_{i=1}^{8} (\pi_i \cdot \pi_i) - \sum_{i=1}^{8} \pi_i \sum_{i=1}^{8} \pi_i$$
$$= 8(5.64) - (5.45)(5.45) = 15.42 \qquad \text{(II.11)}$$

$$a_{12} = 8 \sum_{i=1}^{8} (\pi_i \cdot \sigma_i) - \sum_{i=1}^{8} \pi_i \sum_{i=1}^{8} \sigma_i$$
$$= 8(5.30) - (5.45)(6.10) = 9.16 \qquad \text{(II.12)}$$

$$a_{22} = 8 \sum_{i=1}^{8} (\sigma_i \cdot \sigma_i) - \sum_{i=1}^{8} (\sigma_i) \sum_{i=1}^{8} (\sigma_i)$$
$$= 8(602) - (6.10)(6.10) = 10.95 \qquad \text{(II.13)}$$

The elements of matrix C are then determined by substituting into Equation II.9 as shown in Equations II.14 and II.15. The final "c matrix" is given in Equation II.16.

$$c_1 = 8 \sum_{i=1}^{8} (\pi_i y_i) - \sum_{i=1}^{8} \pi_i \sum_{i=1}^{8} y_i$$
$$= 8(29.26) - (5.45)(39.46) = 19.02 \qquad \text{(II.14)}$$

$$c_2 = 8 \sum_{i=1}^{8} (\sigma_i y_i) - \sum_{i=1}^{8} \sigma_i \sum_{i=1}^{8} y_i$$
$$= 8(33.36) - (6.10)(39.46) = 26.17 \qquad \text{(II.15)}$$

$$\begin{bmatrix} 19.02 \\ 26.17 \end{bmatrix} \qquad \text{(II.16)}$$

From these matrices, one is then able to obtain the final solution. From Equation II.7, it may be shown that the partial regression coefficients (a, b) may be determined from elements of the constant term matrix B and the elements of the inverse of matrix A, the coefficients of the normal equations. Matrix A may be inverted by any of several methods such as the "rolling inverse method" used in the computer program in Appendix III. Since the matrix in our hypothetical model is a 2 X 2 matrix, it may be easily inverted according to Equation II.17 in which a, b, c, and d represent the elements of the matrix and D represents the determinant of matrix D (D = ad - bc).

$$\underset{\underline{D}}{\begin{bmatrix} a & b \\ c & d \end{bmatrix}} = \underset{\underline{E}}{\begin{bmatrix} d/D & -b/D \\ -c/D & a/D \end{bmatrix}} \quad \text{(II.17)}$$

Thus, the inverse of matrix II.10 in our example becomes E as shown in Equation II.18.

$$\underset{D}{\begin{bmatrix} 15.42 & 9.15 \\ 9.15 & 10.95 \end{bmatrix}^{-1}} = \underset{E}{\begin{bmatrix} 10.95/85.12 & -9.15/85.12 \\ -9.15/85.12 & 15.42/85.12 \end{bmatrix}} = \underset{\underline{F}}{\begin{bmatrix} 0.129 & -0.108 \\ -0.108 & 0.182 \end{bmatrix}} \quad \text{(II.18)}$$

If the elements of this inverse matrix (F) are denoted by e_{hj} (h = 1, ... k: j = 1,2... k) then the solution of the partial regression coefficients may be represented by Equation II.19:

$$b_j = \sum_{h=1}^{k} c_h \, e_{hj} \qquad (j = 1,\ 2) \qquad \text{(II.19)}$$

Substitution into Equation II.19 yields the values of a and b for Equation 4.1. This is represented by solution of Equations II.20 and II.21 for a and b, respectively:

$$a = b_1 = \sum_{h=1}^{2} c_h \, e_{h1} = (19.02)(0.129) + (26.17)(-0.108) = -0.373 \qquad \text{(II.20)}$$

$$b = b_2 = \sum_{h=1}^{2} c_h \, e_{h2} = (19.02)(-0.108) + (26.17)(0.182) = 2.709 \qquad \text{(II.21)}$$

The constant of the regression, c (4.1) may then be obtained by substituting into Equation II.22,

$$c = \bar{y} - b_1\bar{x}_1 - b_2\bar{x}_2 . \ . \ . - b_k\bar{x}_k \qquad \text{(II.22)}$$

where $\bar{y}$ is the mean value of y, $\bar{y} = (\sum_{i=1}^{n} yi)/n$, and $\bar{x}_1$, $\bar{x}_2$, . . . $\bar{x}_k$ represent the mean values of the independent variables. Substituting into Equation II.22 for the values from our hypothetical model yields Equation II.23:

$$c = \left(\frac{\sum_{i=1}^{8} y_i}{8}\right) - (-0.373)\left(\frac{\sum_{i=1}^{8} \pi_i}{8}\right) - (2.709)\left(\sum_{i=1}^{8} \frac{\sigma_i}{8}\right)$$

$$= (4.933) - (-0.373)(0.681) - (2.709)(0.763)$$

$$= 3.120 \qquad \text{(II.23)}$$

This completes the least squares solution of the linear equations (4.2-4.9) with the generation of all three constants (a, b, c) in these equations.

APPENDIX III

LINEAR FREE ANALYSIS RELATED PROGRESS FOR SINGLE AND MULTIPLE LINEAR REGRESSION ANALYSES. PROGRAM LISTING, SAMPLE INPUT, AND SAMPLE OUTPUT

```
C       SINGLE AND MULTIPLE LINEAR REGRESSION
C
C       INPUT
C          1) 3 CARDS OF ALPHABETIC INFORMATION
C          2) 1 CARD INDICATING IF TRANSFORMATIONS ARE DESIRED ON THE
C             DEPENDENT VARIABLE(FORMAT(I2))
C             A -1 INDICATES THAT THE NEGATIVE VALUES OF THE LOGS OF THE
C             DEPENDENT VARIABLES ARE TO BE USED,
C             A +1 INDICATES THAT THE POSITIVE VALUES OF THE LOGS OF THE
C             DEPENDENT VARIABLES ARE TO BE USED,
C             00 INDICATES THAT NO TRANSFORMATIONS ARE NECESSARY
C          3)1 CARD WITH
C                   K = TOTAL NO. OF VARIABLES AVAILABLE FOR ANALYSIS
C                       (COLS. 1-2)
C                   N = NO. OF DATA POINTS  (COLS. 3-6)
C                   NRMX = TOTAL NO. OF RUNS FOR THIS ANALYSIS (COLS. 7-10)
C                       (FORMAT-I2,2I4)
C          4)A TOTAL OF K CARDS WITH VARIABLE NO. PUNCHED IN COLS. 1-2
C                   AND VARIABLE NAME PUNCHED IN COLS. 4-15
C          5)DATA CARDS - A SERIES OF CARDS   WITH THE DEPENDENT VARIABLE
C                   FOR EACH EQUATION ON THE FIRST CARD(FORMAT-F7.4)
C                   AND THE INDEPENDENT VARIABLE(S) FOR THAT EQUATION ON THE
C                   NEXT CARD(S)(FORMAT -10F7.4)
C                   THERE SHOULD BE N SERIES OF THESE CARDS
C          6) A SERIES OF NRMX CARDS, EACH OF WHICH INDICATES THE IND.
C                   VARIABLES TO BE USED FOR THIS ANALYSIS (FORMAT 10I1)
C                   A 1 INDICATES THAT THE VARIABLE IS TO BE USED FOR THIS
C                   ANALYSIS AND A 0 INDICATES IT IS NOT TO BE USED FOR THIS
C                   ANALYSIS
C       MAXIMUM NO. OF INDEPENDENT VARIABLES = 10
C       MAXIMUM NO. OF EQUATIONS (DATA POINTS)= 75
C       MAXIMUM NO. OF RUNS = 40
        DIMENSION A(10,10),C(10),SUMX(10),SUMXY(10),W(10),KV(10,40),
       1V(75,10),Y(75),T(10),RMS(40),EXPV(40),F(40),AL(60),FIDENT(10,3),
       2IDF(2,40)
C       ICR=CARD READER
C       LP=LINE PRINER
        ICR= 1
        LP = 3
        WRITE (LP,499)
499     FORMAT(38H1SINGLE AND MULTIPLE LINEAR REGRESSION)
C       READ 3 CARDS OF ALPHABETIC INFORMATION
        READ (ICR,500) AL
500     FORMAT(20A4)
        WRITE (LP,505) AL
505     FORMAT(1H0,20A4/(1H ,20A4))
C
C       IND = -1,0, OR 1 (INDICATES IF LOG IS TO BE TAKEN)
C
        READ (ICR,515) IND
515     FORMAT(I2)
C
C       READ IN NO. OF VARIABLES,NO. OF DATA POINTS, AND NO. OF RUNS
C
        READ (ICR,520) EK, EN,NRMX
520     FORMAT (F2.0,F4.0,I4)
C
```

```
C      READ IN VARIABLE NOS. AND NAMES
       WRITE (LP,522)
       K= IFIX(EK)
       N = IFIX (EN)
       NRUN=0
       SUMY=0.
       SUMYS=0.
       NL = 7
       DO 10 I=1,K
       READ (ICR,525) J,(FIDENT(J,L),L=1,3)
525    FORMAT(I2,1X,3A4)
10     WRITE (LP,530) J,(FIDENT(J,L),L=1,3)
530    FORMAT(1H ,I2,1X,3A4)
522    FORMAT(38HOVARIABLES AVAILABLE FOR THIS ANALYSIS)
C
C      READ Y-X(I) DATA IN AND CHECK FOR DUPLICATE ENTRIES
C
       NL = NL + K + 2
       WRITE (LP,532)
532    FORMAT (11HOINPUT DATA)
       NL1 = (K+7)/8
       DO 35 I=1,N
       READ (ICR,535) Y(I)
       READ (ICR,535) (V(I,J),J=1,K)
535    FORMAT(10F7.4)
       WRITE (LP,540) Y(I)
540    FORMAT(11HOACTIVITY =,F10.4,10X,28HINDEPENDENT VARIABLES FOLLOW)
       WRITE (LP,545)(V(I,J),J=1,K)
       NL = NL+ NL1 + 2
       IF (NL-50) 19,17,17
17     NL = 0
       WRITE (LP,546)
546    FORMAT(1H1)
545    FORMAT(8F10.4)
19     IF(I-1)35,35,20
20     M = I-1
       DO 33 KN=1,M
       IF (Y(I)-Y(KN)) 35,25,35
25     DO 30 J=1,K
       IF (V(I,J)-V(KN,J)) 35,30,35
30     CONTINUE
       WRITE (LP,550) I,KN
550    FORMAT(33HOERROR-DUPLICATE ENTRIES-EQUATION,I4,11H = EQUATION,
      1I4)
32     CALL EXIT
33     CONTINUE
35     CONTINUE
C
       IF (IND)40,60,50
40     WRITE (LP,555)
555    FORMAT(45HONEGATIVES OF THE LOGS OF THE ACTIVITIES USED)
       DO 45 I=1,N
45     Y(I)= -ALOG10(Y(I))
       GO TO 60
50     WRITE (LP,560)
560    FORMAT(51HOPOSITIVE VALUES OF THE LOGS OF THE ACTIVITIES USED)
       DO 55 I=1,N
```

```
55      Y(I)=ALOG10(Y(I))
C
C       SUMMATION OF Y AND Y**2
C
60      DO 65 I =1,N
        SUMY=SUMY +Y(I)
65      SUMYS = SUMYS + Y(I)*Y(I)
C
C       READ IN CARD INDICATING WHICH VARIABLES TO USE IN THIS EQUATION
67      NRUN=NRUN+1
        READ (ICR,565) (KV(I,NRUN),I=1,K)
        KNT = 0
565     FORMAT(10I1)
        WRITE (LP,566) AL
566     FORMAT(1H1,20A4/(1H ,20A4))
        WRITE (LP,570)NRUN
570     FORMAT(27H0VARIABLES USED FOR RUN NO.,I3)
        NL=6
        DO 75 I = 1,K
        IF(KV(I,NRUN)) 75,75,70
70      KNT = KNT +1
        WRITE (LP,575) (FIDENT(I,J),J=1,3)
575     FORMAT(5X,3A4)
75      CONTINUE
        NL=NL+KNT+6
C
C       KNT = NO. OF VARIABLES USED IN THIS REGRESSION
C
        WRITE (LP,580) KNT
580     FORMAT(10X,53HNO. OF INDEPENDENT VARIABLES USED IN THIS REGRESSION
       1=,I3)
        WRITE (LP,581) N
581     FORMAT(10X,20HNO. OF DATA POINTS =,I4)
        EKNT= FLOAT(KNT)
        DO 80 L =1,KNT
        SUMX(L)=0.0
        SUMXY(L)=0.0
        DO 80 J = L,KNT
80      A(L,J) = 0.0
        DO 95 I=1,N
        L=0
        DO 90 M = 1,K
        IF (KV(M,NRUN)) 90,90,85
85      L = L+1
        W(L) =V(I,M)
90      CONTINUE
        DO 95 L = 1,KNT
        SUMX(L) = SUMX(L) + W(L)
        SUMXY(L) = SUMXY(L) + W(L)*Y(I)
        DO 95 J = L,KNT
95      A(L,J) = A(L,J) + W(L) * W(J)
C
C       COMPUTE COFFICIENT OF VARIATION (STANDARD DEVIATION * 100/
C       THE MEAN)
        DO 105 L = 1,KNT
        DSQ = (A(L,L) - SUMX(L)*SUMX(L)/EN)/(EN-1.0)
        D = SQRT(DSQ)
```

```
      CV = (D*100.)/(SUMX(L)/EN)
      CV = ABS(CV)
      IF (CV - .25) 100,100,105
100   IF (CV) 102,101,102
101   WRITE (LP,582) L
582   FORMAT(44HOCOEFFICIENT OF VARIATION = 0.0 FOR VARIABLE,I3/
     1 18H THIS RUN SKIPPED.)
      NRUN = NRUN - 1
      NRMX = NRMX - 1
      GO TO 181
102   WRITE (LP, 585) L,CV
585   FORMAT (48HO***** THE COEFFICIENT OF VARIATION FOR VARIABLE,I3,
     114H IN THIS RUN =,E14.8/7X,32HILL CONDITIONING MAY BE A FACTOR)
105   CONTINUE
      DO 110 L = 1,KNT
      C(L)=EN*SUMXY(L)-SUMX(L)*SUMY
      DO 110 J = L,KNT
      A(L,J) = EN*A(L,J) - SUMX(L) * SUMX(J)
110   A(J,L) = A(L,J)
      WRITE (LP,590)
590   FORMAT(38HOCORRELATION COEFFICIENTS X(L) TO X(J) /
     1 1HO,8X,1HL,9X,1HJ,11X,6HR(L,J))
      DO 115 L = 1,KNT
      DO 115 J = L,KNT
      R=A(L,J)/SQRT (A(L,L)*A(J,J))
      NL=NL+1
      IF(NL-50)115,113,113
113   NL=0
      WRITE(LP,546)
115   WRITE (LP,595) L,J,R
595   FORMAT(2I10,E20.8)
C     MATRIX INVERSION
      K1 = KNT - 1
      IF (K1) 32,120,125
120   A(1,1) = 1.0/A(1,1)
      GO TO 150
125   DO 145 ITER = 1,KNT
      W(KNT) = 1.0/A(1,1)
      DO 130 J=1,K1
130   W(J)=A(1,J+1)*W(KNT)
      DO 140 L =1,K1
      DO 135 J =1,K1
135   A(L,J) =A(L+1,J+1)-A(L+1,1) *W(J)
140   A(L,KNT)= -A(L+1,1)*W(KNT)
      DO 145 J=1,KNT
145   A(KNT,J) = W(J)
C
C     COMPUTATION OF REGRESSION COEFFICIENTS
C
150   SUM=0.0
      BZERO = SUMY/EN
      DO 160 J = 1,KNT
      W(J)=0.0
      DO 155 L=1,KNT
155   W(J)=W(J)+ C(L)*A(L,J)
      SUM=SUM+W(J)*C(J)
160   BZERO=BZERO - W(J)*SUMX(J)/EN
```

```
      WRITE (LP,600)
600   FORMAT(24HOREGRESSION COEFFICIENTS /
     1 1HO,18X, 1HJ, 11X, 5H B(J))
      J=0
      WRITE (LP,605) J,BZERO
605   FORMAT(10X,I10,E20.8)
      DO 165 J=1,KNT
165   WRITE (LP,605)  J, W(J)
C
C     COMPUTATION OF THE MULTIPLE CORRELATION COEFFICIENT
C     COMPUTATION OF THE STANDARD ERROR OF THE Y DATA
C     COMPUTATION OF THE STANDARD ERROR OF THE ESTIMATE
C     COMPUTATION CF THE SIGNIFICANCE OF REGRESSION (F)
C     COMPUTATION OF THE EXPLAINED VARIANCE
C
      NL=NL+18+KNT
      IF(NL-54)167,166,166
166   NL=0
      WRITE(LP,546)
167   IR=NRUN
      AYY= EN*SUMYS -SUMY*SUMY
      RMS(IR) = SUM/AYY
      SY = AYY/(EN*(EN-1.))
      SYX= SY*(EN-1.0)*(1.0-RMS(IR))/(EN-EKNT-1.0)
      F(IR) =SUM/(EN*EKNT*SYX)
      EXPV(IR) = 1.0 -(SYX/SY)
      RMULT= SQRT(RMS(IR))
      IDF(1,IR)=KNT
      IDF(2,IR)=N-1-KNT
      SY=SQRT(SY)
      SYX=SQRT(SYX)
      WRITE(LP,610) RMULT
610   FORMAT(1HO/35H MULTIPLE CORRELATION COEFFICIENT =,E20.8)
      WRITE (LP,615) RMS(IR)
615   FORMAT(1HO,25X,9HR ** 2 = ,E20.8)
      WRITE (LP,620) SY
620   FORMAT(35HOSTANDARD ERROR OF THE Y DATA     =,E20.8)
      WRITE (LP,625) SYX
625   FORMAT(35HOSTANDARD ERROR OF THE ESTIMATE   =,E20:8)
      WRITE (LP,630) F(IR), IDF(1,IR),IDF(2,IR)
630   FORMAT(35HOSIGNFICANCE OF REGRESSION (F)    =,E20.8,5X,6HD.F. =,
     1I3,4H AND,I4)
      WRITE (LP,635) EXPV(IR)
635   FORMAT(35HOAMCUNT OF EXPLAINED VARIANCE     =,E20.8//)
C
C     COMPUTATION OF THE STANDARD ERROR OF THE PARTIAL REGRESSION
C     COEFFICIENTS AND THE T VALUE FOR INDIVIDUAL COEFFICIENT
C     SIGNIFICANCE
      NL=NL+5+KNT
      IF(NL-54)169,169,168
168   NL=0
      WRITE(LP,546)
169   WRITE (LP,640)
640   FORMAT(50HOSTANDARD ERROR OF PARTIAL REGRESSION COEFFICIENTS/
     1 1HO,17X,2H J,10X,6H SB(J))
      SB=1.0
      DO 170 L=1,KNT
```

```
      DO 170 J=1,KNT
170   SB=SB+A(L,J)*SUMX(L)*SUMX(J)
      SB=SYX*SQRT (SB/EN)
      J=0
      WRITE (LP,605) J,SB
      DO 175 J=1,KNT
      SB=SYX*SQRT (EN*A(J,J))
      T(J)=W(J)/SB
175   WRITE(LP,605) J,SB
      NL=NL+3+KNT
      IF(NL-54)177,177,176
176   NL=0
      WRITE(LP,546)
177   WRITE (LP,645)
645   FORMAT(38HOT VALUES FOR COEFFICIENT SIGNIFICANCE/)
      DO 180 J=1,KNT
180   WRITE (LP,650) J,T(J)
650   FORMAT(10X,2HT(,I2,3H) =,F15.8)
181   IF(NRUN-NRMX)67,185,185
185   WRITE(LP,655)
655   FORMAT(20H1SUMMARY OF ANALYSES///
     14H RUN,6X,15HPARAMETERS USED,6X,4HR**2,3X,9HEXPLAINED,5X,1HF,
     211X,2HDF /38X,8HVARIANCE)
      DO 250 IR=1,NRUN
      DO 195 I=1,K
      IF(KV(I,IR))200 ,195,200
195   CONTINUE
200   WRITE (LP,660) IR,(FIDENT(I,J),J=1,3),RMS(IR),EXPV(IR),F(IR),
     1 IDF(1,IR),IDF(2,IR)
660   FORMAT(1H0,I3,6X,3A4,F13.3,F10.3,F11.3,I6,4H AND,I4)
      IF (I-K) 205,250,250
205   M=I+1
      DO  215 I=M,K
      IF(KV(I,IR))215,215,210
210   WRITE (LP,665)(FIDENT(I,J),J=1,3)
665   FORMAT (10X,3A4)
215   CONTINUE
250   CONTINUE
      CALL EXIT
      END
  END OF DATA
```

```
CARIES PILOT PROJECT  1-5-71
MONOAMINE HYDROFLUORIDES VS STREP FAECALIS
TURBIDIMETRIC GROWTH INHIBITION STUDIES  --  ALL DODECYL  --  C12
-1
06   9  11
01 PI2
02 PI
03 PI-HEAD
04 PI-TAIL
05 QN
06 ES
3.1
17.222504.15  -1.85   6.00   0.131  2.48
2.8
21.160004.60  -1.40   6.00  00.433 01.24
2.55
26.0100 5.10  -0.90   6.00   0.431  1.17
3.13
31.6969 5.63  -0.37  06.00  04.28  -0.30
6.0
25.2025 5.05  -0.95   6.00  00.692 00.0
3.57
36.6025 6.05  00.05   6.00   0.686 -0.14
100.0
93.1225 9.65   3.65   6.00   0.685 -1.86
3.45
44.2225 6.65   0.65   6.00   0.685 -0.94
2.30
49.7025 7.05   1.05   6.00   0.685 -0.46
010000
001000
000010
000001
110000
010010
010001
010011
110010
110001
110011
 END OF DATA
```

```
SINGLE AND MULTIPLE LINEAR REGRESSION

CARIES PILOT PROJECT  1-5-71
MONOAMINE HYDROFLUORIDES VS STREP FAECALIS
TURBIDIMETRIC GROWTH INHIBITION STUDIES  --  ALL DODECYL  --  C12

VARIABLES AVAILABLE FOR THIS ANALYSIS
 1 PI2
 2 PI
 3 PI-HEAD
 4 PI-TAIL
 5 QN
 6 ES

INPUT DATA

ACTIVITY =     3.1000             INDEPENDENT VARIABLES FOLLOW
  17.2225    4.1500   -1.8500   6.0000    0.1310    2.4800

ACTIVITY =     2.8000             INDEPENDENT VARIABLES FOLLOW
  21.1600    4.6000   -1.4000   6.0000    0.4330    1.2400

ACTIVITY =     2.5500             INDEPENDENT VARIABLES FOLLOW
  26.0100    5.1000   -0.9000   6.0000    0.4310    1.1700

ACTIVITY =     3.1300             INDEPENDENT VARIABLES FOLLOW
  31.6969    5.6300   -0.3700   6.0000    4.2800   -0.3000

ACTIVITY =     6.0000             INDEPENDENT VARIABLES FOLLOW
  25.2025    5.0500   -0.9500   6.0000    0.6920    0.0

ACTIVITY =     3.5700             INDEPENDENT VARIABLES FOLLOW
  36.6025    6.0500    0.0500   6.0000    0.6860   -0.1400

ACTIVITY =   100.0000             INDEPENDENT VARIABLES FOLLOW
  93.1225    9.6500    3.6500   6.0000    0.6850   -1.8600

ACTIVITY =     3.4500             INDEPENDENT VARIABLES FOLLOW
  44.2225    6.6500    0.6500   6.0000    0.6850   -0.9400

ACTIVITY =     2.3000             INDEPENDENT VARIABLES FOLLOW
  49.7025    7.0500    1.0500   6.0000    0.6850   -0.4600

NEGATIVES OF THE LOGS OF THE ACTIVITIES USED
```

```
CARIES PILOT PROJECT  1-5-71
MONOAMINE HYDROFLUORIDES VS STREP FAECALIS
TURBIDIMETRIC GROWTH INHIBITION STUDIES  --  ALL DODECYL  --  C12

VARIABLES USED FOR RUN NO.  1
    PI
          NO. OF INDEPENDENT VARIABLES USED IN THIS REGRESSION=  1
          NO. OF DATA POINTS =    9

CORRELATION COEFFICIENTS X(L) TO X(J)

       L          J            R(L,J)
       1          1       0.10000000E 01

REGRESSION COEFFICIENTS

                  J            B(J)
                  0       0.75846577E 00
                  1      -0.23914659E 00


MULTIPLE CORRELATION COEFFICIENT =        0.77768558E 00

                        R ** 2 =          0.60479486E 00

STANDARD ERROR OF THE Y DATA      =       0.51089329E 00

STANDARD ERROR OF THE ESTIMATE    =       0.34335023E 00

SIGNFICANCE OF REGRESSION (F)     =       0.10712324E 02     D.F. =  1 AND   7

AMOUNT OF EXPLAINED VARIANCE      =       0.54833716E 00


STANDARD ERROR OF PARTIAL REGRESSION COEFFICIENTS

                  J            SB(J)
                  0       0.45254564E 00
                  1       0.73067129E-01

T VALUES FOR COEFFICIENT SIGNIFICANCE

          T( 1) =    -3.27297020
```

```
CARIES PILOT PROJECT  1-5-71
MONOAMINE HYDROFLUORIDES VS STREP FAECALIS
TURBIDIMETRIC GROWTH INHIBITION STUDIES  --  ALL DODECYL  --  C12

VARIABLES USED FOR RUN NO.  2
    PI-HEAD
         NO. OF INDEPENDENT VARIABLES USED IN THIS REGRESSION=  1
         NO. OF DATA POINTS =    9

CORRELATION COEFFICIENTS X(L) TO X(J)

        L          J            R(L,J)
        1          1       0.10000000E 01

REGRESSION COEFFICIENTS

                   J            B(J)
                   0      -0.67641193E 00
                   1      -0.23914886E 00


MULTIPLE CORRELATION COEFFICIENT =       0.77768862E 00

                        R ** 2 =         0.60479963E 00

STANDARD ERROR OF THE Y DATA      =      0.51089329E 00

STANDARD ERROR OF THE ESTIMATE    =      0.34334815E 00

SIGNFICANCE OF REGRESSION (F)     =      0.10712543E 02     D.F. =  1 AND   7

AMOUNT OF EXPLAINED VARIANCE      =      0.54834265E 00


STANDARD ERROR OF PARTIAL REGRESSION COEFFICIENTS

                   J           SB(J)
                   0       0.11445069E 00
                   1       0.73067069E-01

T VALUES FOR COEFFICIENT SIGNIFICANCE

         T( 1) =      -3.27300453
```

```
CARIES PILOT PROJECT  1-5-71
MONOAMINE HYDROFLUORIDES VS STREP FAECALIS
TURBIDIMETRIC GROWTH INHIBITION STUDIES  --  ALL DODECYL  --  C12

VARIABLES USED FOR RUN NO.  3
    QN
         NO. OF INDEPENDENT VARIABLES USED IN THIS REGRESSION=  1
         NO. OF DATA POINTS =    9

CORRELATION COEFFICIENTS X(L) TO X(J)

        L          J            R(L,J)
        1          1       0.10000000E 01

REGRESSION COEFFICIENTS

                   J            B(J)
                   0       -0.70639956E 00
                   1        0.32915551E-01


MULTIPLE CORRELATION COEFFICIENT =        0.80985367E-01

                         R ** 2 =         0.65586306E-02

STANDARD ERROR OF THE Y DATA       =      0.51089329E 00

STANDARD ERROR OF THE ESTIMATE     =      0.54437381E 00

SIGNFICANCE OF REGRESSION (F)      =      0.46213545E-01     D.F. =  1 AND   7

AMOUNT OF EXPLAINED VARIANCE       =     -0.13536072E 00


STANDARD ERROR OF PARTIAL REGRESSION COEFFICIENTS

                   J           SB(J)
                   0       0.23425287E 00
                   1       0.15311450E 00

T VALUES FOR COEFFICIENT SIGNIFICANCE

         T( 1) =     0.21497339
```

```
CARIES PILOT PROJECT  1-5-71
MONOAMINE HYDROFLUORIDES VS STREP FAECALIS
TURBIDIMETRIC GROWTH INHIBITION STUDIES  --  ALL DODECYL  --  C12

VARIABLES USED FOR RUN NO.  4
    ES
         NO. OF INDEPENDENT VARIABLES USED IN THIS REGRESSION=  1
         NO. OF DATA POINTS =    9

CORRELATION COEFFICIENTS X(L) TO X(J)

        L          J           R(L,J)
        1          1       0.10000000E 01

REGRESSION COEFFICIENTS

                   J           B(J)
                   0      -0.70547265E 00
                   1       0.23385453E 00


MULTIPLE CORRELATION COEFFICIENT =       0.59602374E 00

                         R ** 2 =       0.35524434E 00

STANDARD ERROR OF THE Y DATA      =       0.51089329E 00

STANDARD ERROR OF THE ESTIMATE    =       0.43855447E 00

SIGNFICANCE OF REGRESSION (F)     =       0.38568287E 01      D.F. =  1 AND   7

AMOUNT OF EXPLAINED VARIANCE      =       0.26313698E 00


STANDARD ERROR OF PARTIAL REGRESSION COEFFICIENTS

                   J           SB(J)
                   0       0.14703017E 00
                   1       0.11907768E 00

T VALUES FOR COEFFICIENT SIGNIFICANCE

         T( 1) =     1.96388149
```

```
CARIES PILOT PROJECT  1-5-71
MONOAMINE HYDROFLUORIDES VS STREP FAECALIS
TURBIDIMETRIC GROWTH INHIBITION STUDIES  --  ALL DODECYL  --  C12

VARIABLES USED FOR RUN NO.  5
    PI2
    PI
         NO. OF INDEPENDENT VARIABLES USED IN THIS REGRESSION=  2
         NO. OF DATA POINTS =    9

CORRELATION COEFFICIENTS X(L) TC X(J)

        L          J            R(L,J)
        1          1       0.10000000E 01
        1          2       0.99166417E 00
        2          2       0.10000000E 01

REGRESSION COEFFICIENTS

                   J             B(J)
                   0      -0.32939024E 01
                   1      -0.91308594E-01
                   2       0.10211449E 01


MULTIPLE CORRELATION COEFFICIENT =          0.94251889E 00

                           R ** 2 =         0.88834196E 00

STANDARD ERROR OF THE Y DATA       =        0.51089329E 00

STANDARD ERROR OF THE ESTIMATE     =        0.19712627E 00

SIGNFICANCE OF REGRESSION (F)      =        0.23867752E 02      D.F. =  2 AND   6

AMOUNT OF EXPLAINED VARIANCE       =        0.85112268E C0


STANDARD ERROR OF PARTIAL REGRESSION COEFFICIENTS

                   J             SB(J)
                   0       0.10701132E 01
                   1       0.23390889E-01
                   2       0.32556486E 00

T VALUES FOR COEFFICIENT SIGNIFICANCE

         T( 1) =    -3.90359592
         T( 2) =     3.13653278
```

```
CARIES PILOT PROJECT  1-5-71
MONOAMINE HYDROFLUORIDES VS STREP FAECALIS
TURBIDIMETRIC GROWTH INHIBITION STUDIES  --  ALL DODECYL  --  C12

VARIABLES USED FOR RUN NO.  6
    PI
    QN
         NO. OF INDEPENDENT VARIABLES USED IN THIS REGRESSION=  2
         NO. OF DATA POINTS =    9

CORRELATION COEFFICIENTS X(L) TO X(J)

        L         J           R(L,J)
        1         1       0.10000000E 01
        1         2       0.17318226E-01
        2         2       0.10000000E 01

REGRESSION COEFFICIENTS

                  J            B(J)
                  0       0.72432518E 00
                  1      -0.23964971E 00
                  2       0.38401034E-01


MULTIPLE CORRELATION COEFFICIENT =        0.78340209E 00

                          R ** 2 =        0.61371887E 00

STANDARD ERROR OF THE Y DATA      =       0.51089329E 00

STANDARD ERROR OF THE ESTIMATE    =       0.36664963E 00

SIGNFICANCE OF REGRESSION (F)     =       0.47663660E 01      D.F. =  2 AND   6

AMOUNT OF EXPLAINED VARIANCE      =       0.48495865E 00


STANDARD ERROR OF PARTIAL REGRESSION COEFFICIENTS

                  J            SB(J)
                  0       0.49187768E 00
                  1       0.78037083E-01
                  2       0.10314196E 00

T VALUES FOR COEFFICIENT SIGNIFICANCE

         T( 1) =     -3.07097149
         T( 2) =      0.37231237
```

```
CARIES PILOT PROJECT  1-5-71
MONOAMINE HYDROFLUORIDES VS STREP FAECALIS
TURBIDIMETRIC GROWTH INHIBITION STUDIES  --  ALL DODECYL  --  C12

VARIABLES USED FOR RUN NO.  7
    PI
    ES
         NO. OF INDEPENDENT VARIABLES USED IN THIS REGRESSION=  2
         NO. OF DATA POINTS =    9

CORRELATION COEFFICIENTS X(L) TO X(J)

       L         J          R(L,J)
       1         1      0.10000000E 01
       1         2     -0.87520790E 00
       2         2      0.10000000E 01

REGRESSION COEFFICIENTS

                 J          B(J)
                 0      0.13603344E 01
                 1     -0.33645833E 00
                 2     -0.14186591E 00

MULTIPLE CORRELATION COEFFICIENT =        0.79711193E 00

                        R ** 2 =          0.63538742E 00

STANDARD ERROR OF THE Y DATA      =       0.51089329E 00

STANDARD ERROR OF THE ESTIMATE    =       0.35621756E 00

SIGNFICANCE OF REGRESSION (F)     =       0.52279139E 01     D.F. =  2 AND   6

AMOUNT OF EXPLAINED VARIANCE      =       0.51385003E 00


STANDARD ERROR OF PARTIAL REGRESSION COEFFICIENTS

                 J          SB(J)
                 0      0.96952808E 00
                 1      0.15670443E 00
                 2      0.19994169E 00

T VALUES FOR COEFFICIENT SIGNIFICANCE

        T( 1) =    -2.14708805
        T( 2) =    -0.70953637
```

```
CARIES PILOT PROJECT  1-5-71
MONOAMINE HYDROFLUORIDES VS STREP FAECALIS
TURBIDIMETRIC GROWTH INHIBITION STUDIES  --  ALL DODECYL  --  C12

VARIABLES USED FOR RUN NO.   8
    PI
    QN
    ES
         NO. OF INDEPENDENT VARIABLES USED IN THIS REGRESSION=  3
         NO. OF DATA POINTS =    9

CORRELATION COEFFICIENTS X(L) TO X(J)

        L           J            R(L,J)
        1           1        0.10000000E 01
        1           2        0.17318226E-01
        1           3       -0.87520790E 00
        2           2        0.10000000E 01
        2           3       -0.25954217E 00
        3           3        0.10000000E 01

REGRESSION COEFFICIENTS

                    J             B(J)
                    0        0.13431520E 01
                    1       -0.33420169E 00
                    2        0.33249855E-02
                    3       -0.13851357E 00

MULTIPLE CORRELATION COEFFICIENT =          0.79714203E 00

                            R ** 2 =        0.63543546E 00

STANDARD ERROR OF THE Y DATA       =        0.51089329E 00

STANDARD ERROR OF THE ESTIMATE     =        0.39019108E 00

SIGNFICANCE OF REGRESSION (F)      =        0.29049978E 01     D.F. =  3 AND   5

AMOUNT OF EXPLAINED VARIANCE       =        0.41669691E 00


STANDARD ERROR OF PARTIAL REGRESSION COEFFICIENTS

                    J             SB(J)
                    0        0.12488480E 01
                    1        0.19212008E 00
                    2        0.12719476E 00
                    3        0.25378931E 00
```

```
T VALUES FOR COEFFICIENT SIGNIFICANCE

         T( 1) =    -1.73954582
         T( 2) =     0.02614090
         T( 3) =    -0.54578167

CARIES PILOT PROJECT  1-5-71
MONOAMINE HYDROFLUORIDES VS STREP FAECALIS
TURBIDIMETRIC GROWTH INHIBITION STUDIES  --  ALL DODECYL  --  C12

VARIABLES USED FOR RUN NO.  9
    PI2
    PI
    QN
        NO. OF INDEPENDENT VARIABLES USED IN THIS REGRESSION=  3
        NO. OF DATA POINTS =   9

CORRELATION COEFFICIENTS X(L) TO X(J)

        L          J           R(L,J)
        1          1       0.10000000E 01
        1          2       0.99166417E 00
        1          3      -0.20565014E-01
        2          2       0.10000000E 01
        2          3       0.17318226E-01
        3          3       0.10000000E 01

REGRESSION COEFFICIENTS

                   J           B(J)
                   0      -0.34195089E 01
                   1      -0.94689071E-01
                   2       0.10681458E 01
                   3      -0.27356405E-01

MULTIPLE CORRELATION COEFFICIENT =        0.94473547E 00

                          R ** 2 =        0.89252514E 00

STANDARD ERROR OF THE Y DATA      =       0.51089329E 00

STANDARD ERROR OF THE ESTIMATE    =       0.21185738E 00

SIGNFICANCE OF REGRESSION (F)     =       0.13840849E 02     D.F. =  3 AND   5

AMOUNT OF EXPLAINED VARIANCE      =       0.82804030E 00


STANDARD ERROR OF PARTIAL REGRESSION COEFFICIENTS

                   J          SB(J)
                   0      0.11852026E 01
                   1      0.26292201E-01
                   2      0.36592400E 00
                   3      0.62331699E-01
```

```
T VALUES FOR COEFFICIENT SIGNIFICANCE

        T( 1) =     -3.60141277
        T( 2) =      2.91903687
        T( 3) =     -0.43888426


CARIES PILOT PROJECT  1-5-71
MONOAMINE HYDROFLUORIDES VS STREP FAECALIS
TURBIDIMETRIC GROWTH INHIBITION STUDIES  --  ALL DODECYL  --  C12

VARIABLES USED FOR RUN NO. 10
    PI2
    PI
    ES
        NO. OF INDEPENDENT VARIABLES USED IN THIS REGRESSION=  3
        NO. OF DATA POINTS =    9

CORRELATION COEFFICIENTS X(L) TO X(J)

        L         J          R(L,J)
        1         1      0.10000000E 01
        1         2      0.99166417E 00
        1         3     -0.82406855E 00
        2         2      0.10000000E 01
        2         3     -0.87520790E 00
        3         3      0.10000000E 01

REGRESSION COEFFICIENTS

                  J          B(J)
                  0     -0.67688875E 01
                  1     -0.13897085E 00
                  2      0.18988419E 01
                  3      0.32051945E 00


MULTIPLE CORRELATION COEFFICIENT =          0.98350769E 00

                         R ** 2 =           0.96728748E 00

STANDARD ERROR OF THE Y DATA          =     0.51089329E 00

STANDARD ERROR OF THE ESTIMATE        =     0.11688185E 00

SIGNFICANCE OF REGRESSION (F)         =     0.49282242E 02     D.F. =   3 AND   5

AMOUNT OF EXPLAINED VARIANCE          =     0.94766003E 00


STANDARD ERROR OF PARTIAL REGRESSION COEFFICIENTS

                  J          SB(J)
                  0      0.11848774E 01
                  1      0.19511923E-01
                  2      0.31802785E 00
                  3      0.92296720E-01
```

```
T VALUES FOR COEFFICIENT SIGNIFICANCE

        T( 1) =     -7.12235451
        T( 2) =      5.97067738
        T( 3) =      3.47270679


CARIES PILOT PROJECT  1-5-71
MONOAMINE HYDROFLUORIDES VS STREP FAECALIS
TURBIDIMETRIC GROWTH INHIBITION STUDIES  --  ALL DODECYL  --  C12

VARIABLES USED FOR RUN NO. 11
    PI2
    PI
    QN
    ES
        NO. OF INDEPENDENT VARIABLES USED IN THIS REGRESSION=  4
        NO. OF DATA POINTS =    9

CORRELATION COEFFICIENTS X(L) TO X(J)

        L         J            R(L,J)
        1         1        0.10000000E 01
        1         2        0.99166417E 00
        1         3       -0.20565014E-01
        1         4       -0.82406855E 00
        2         2        0.10000000E 01
        2         3        0.17318226E-01
        2         4       -0.87520790E 00
        3         3        0.10000000E 01
        3         4       -0.25954217E 00
        4         4        0.10000000E 01

REGRESSION COEFFICIENTS

                  J            B(J)
                  0       -0.70259562E 01
                  1       -0.14060253E 00
                  2        0.19463110E 01
                  3        0.31286657E-01
                  4        0.35749054E 00


MULTIPLE CORRELATION COEFFICIENT =       0.98572719E 00

                        R ** 2 =         0.97165817E 00

STANDARD ERROR OF THE Y DATA      =      0.51089329E 00

STANDARD ERROR OF THE ESTIMATE    =      0.12163514E 00

SIGNFICANCE OF REGRESSION (F)     =      0.34283539E 02     D.F. =  4 AND   4

AMOUNT OF EXPLAINED VARIANCE      =      0.94331640E 00
```

STANDARD ERROR OF PARTIAL REGRESSION COEFFICIENTS

J	SB(J)
0	0.12758179E 01
1	0.20411558E-01
2	0.33644170E 00
3	0.39857972E-01
4	0.10697675E 00

T VALUES FOR COEFFICIENT SIGNIFICANCE

T(1) = -6.88837719
T(2) = 5.78498745
T(3) = 0.78495353
T(4) = 3.34175873

SUMMARY OF ANALYSES

RUN	PARAMETERS USED	R**2	EXPLAINED VARIANCE	F	DF
1	PI	0.605	0.548	10.712	1 AND 7
2	PI-HEAD	0.605	0.548	10.713	1 AND 7
3	QN	0.007	-0.135	0.046	1 AND 7
4	ES	0.355	0.263	3.857	1 AND 7
5	PI2 PI	0.888	0.851	23.868	2 AND 6
6	PI QN	0.614	0.485	4.766	2 AND 6
7	PI ES	0.635	0.514	5.228	2 AND 6
8	PI QN ES	0.635	0.417	2.905	3 AND 5
9	PI2 PI QN	0.893	0.828	13.841	3 AND 5
10	PI2 PI ES	0.967	0.948	49.282	3 AND 5
11	PI2 PI QN ES	0.972	0.943	34.284	4 AND 4

APPENDIX IV

DE NOVO, FREE-WILSON PROGRAM. PROGRAM LISTING SAMPLE, INPUT, AND SAMPLE OUTPUT

```
C      FREE-WILSON PROGRAM
C      INPUT
C      CARD 1 - COLS. 1-3 = NRMX= NO. OF RUNS TO BE MADE
C      CARDS 2-5 - ALPHABETIC INFORMATION, PUNCHED IN COLS. 1-80
C      CARD 6
C           COLS. 1-3 = N = NO. OF DATA POINTS = NO. OF EQUATIONS
C           COLS. 4-6 = NRANK = NO. OF VARIABLES
C      BEGIN READING THE N EQUATIONS IN.
C         THE INDEPENDENT VARIABLES ARE FIRST FOLLOWED BY THE DEPENDENT
C         VARIABLE. FORMAT(16F5.0)
C         IF THERE WERE 17 INDEPENDENT VARIABLES AND ONE DEPENDENT
C         VARIABLE, EACH EQUATION WOULD TAKE TWO CARDS, THE FIRST
C         CARD BEING USED FOR IND. VARIABLES 1-16 AND THE SECOND CARD
C         FOR THE 17TH IND. VARIABLE AND FOR THE DEPENDENT VARIABLE.
C
C      THERE IS A MAXIMUM OF 49 INDEPENDENT VARIABLES AND ONE DEPENDENT
C         VARIABLE.
C
C      PROGRAM REQUIRES A MAGNETIC TAPE FOR INTERMEDIATE INPUT/OUTPUT
       DIMENSION A(50,50),V(50),SUM(50),IPVOT(50),INDEX(50,2),PIVOT(50),
      1 FMT(80),C(50),SYM(50),DIAG(50),G(50) , ALPHA1(3),ALPHA2(3)
       EQUIVALENCE (IROW,JROW), (ICOL,JCOL)
C      LP=LINE PRINTER
       LP=3
C      MT=MAGNETIC TAPE
       MT=7
C      ICR=CARD READER
       ICR=1
       READ(ICR,15) NRMX
1      READ (ICR,5) FMT
       WRITE (LP,600) FMT
600    FORMAT(1H1,20A4/(1H ,20A4))
5      FORMAT(20A4)
C
C      N IS THE NO. OF DATA PTS. AND NRANK IS NO. OF VARIABLES USED
C      (INCLUDING DEPENDENT VARIABLE)
C
       READ (ICR,15) N,NRANK
15     FORMAT(2I3)
       FN= FLOAT(N)
       DO 17 I=1,50
17     V(I)=0.0
       DO 20 I=1,NRANK
       SUM(I)=0.0
       DO 20 J=1,NRANK
20     A(I,J)=0.0
       WRITE (LP,18)
18     FORMAT(19H0INPUT DATA FOLLOWS)
C
C      BEGIN READING DATA CARDS AND WRITING THEM ON TAPE
C
       NL=6
       NL1=(MAX+6)/7
       MAX=NRANK-1
       DO 25 I=1,N
       READ (ICR,30) (V(J),J=1,NRANK)
30     FORMAT(16F5.0)
```

```
      WRITE (LP,21) I, V(NRANK)
      NL=NL+2
 21   FORMAT(9H0EQUATION,I5,5X,10HACTIVITY =,F8.3,5X,28HINDEPENDENT VARI
     1ABLES FCLLCW)
      WRITE (LP,22) (V(J),J=1,MAX)
      NL=NL+NL1
      IF(NL-45)25,23,23
 23   NL=0
      WRITE(LP,24)
 24   FORMAT(1H1)
 22   FORMAT(7F10.3)
 25   WRITE (MT) V
      REWIND MT
      DO 35 K=1,N
      READ (MT) V
      KNR=NRANK
C
C     FORM SUMS OF CROSS PRODUCTS FOR MATRIX
C
      DO 35 I =1, KNR
      SUM(I)=SUM(I) + V(I)
      DO 35 J= I, KNR
 35   A(I,J) = A(I,J) + V(I) * V(J)
      REWIND MT
      DO 40 I = 1, KNR
      DO 40 J=  I, KNR
      A(I,J) = A(I,J) - SUM(I) * SUM(J)/FN
 40   A(J,I)= A(I,J)
C     MATRIX INVERSION
C
      MAX = KNR - 1
 45   DET = 1.0
      DO 50  J=1,MAX
 50   IPVOT(J)=0
      DO 110 I=1,MAX
C
C     SEARCH FOR PIVOT ELEMENT
C
      T=0.0
      DO 75 J=1,MAX
      IF(IPVOT(J)-1) 55,75,55
 55   DO 70 K=1,MAX
      IF(IPVOT(K)-1) 60,70,135
 60   IF(ABS(T) - ABS(A(J,K))) 65,70,70
 65   IROW=J
      ICOL=K
      T= A(J,K)
 70   CONTINUE
 75   CONTINUE
      IPVOT(ICOL) = IPVOT(ICOL) + 1
C
C     PLACE PIVOT ELEMENT ON THE DIAGONAL
      IF(IROW - ICOL) 80,90,80
 80   DET = -DET
      DO 85 L= 1,KNR
      T = A(IROW,L)
      A(IROW,L)= A(ICOL,L)
```

```
85     A(ICOL,L) = T
90     INDEX(I,1) = IROW
       INDEX(I,2) = ICOL
       PIVOT(I)= A(ICOL,ICOL)
       DET = DET * PIVOT(I)
C
C      DIVIDE PIVOT ROW BY PIVOT ELEMENT
C
       A(ICOL,ICOL) = 1.0
       DO 95  L= 1, KNR
95     A(ICOL,L) = A(ICOL,L)/PIVOT(I)
C
C      REDUCE NON-PIVOT ROWS
C
       DO 110 LI = 1, MAX
       IF(LI - ICOL) 100,110,100
100    T = A(LI,ICOL)
       A(LI,ICOL) = 0.0
       DO 105 L=1,KNR
105    A(LI,L) = A(LI,L) - A(ICOL,L) * T
110    CONTINUE
C
C      INTERCHANGE COLUMNS
C
115    DO 130 I=1,MAX
       L = MAX - I + 1
       IF(INDEX(L,1) - INDEX(L,2))120,130,120
120    JROW = INDEX(L,1)
       JCOL = INDEX(L,2)
       DO 125 K = 1, MAX
       T = A(K,JROW)
       A(K,JROW) = A(K,JCOL)
       A(K,JCOL) = T
125    CONTINUE
130    CONTINUE
       WRITE (LP,600) FMT
       WRITE(LP,141) N, MAX
141    FORMAT(1H0, I5, 10H COMPOUNDS, 5X, I3, 22H INDEPENDENT VARIABLES)
       WRITE (LP,150) DET
150    FORMAT(28H0VALUE OF THE DETERMINANT = ,E14.8)
155    FORMAT(1H ,I3,1X,E14.8,5X,E14.8)
       NR1 = KNR - 1
       DO 160  I =1, NR1
       C(I)= A(I,KNR)
160    DIAG(I) = A(I,I)
       DO 165  I = 1,KNR
165    SUM(I) = SUM(I)/FN
       F=SUM(KNR)
       DO 170  I = 1,NR1
170    F = F - C(I)*SUM(I)
       I=0
       WRITE (LP,172)   F
172    FORMAT(22H0REGRESSION CONSTANT = ,E14.8/
      1 26H0SUBSTITUENT CONTRIBUTIONS )
       KTOTL = 0
       KCNT = 0
180    READ (ICR,185 ) K , ALPHA1
```

```
185   FORMAT(I3,6X,3A4)
      KCNT= KCNT + 1
190   WRITE (LP,195 ) KCNT
195   FORMAT(6HOGROUP,I3)
      DEPV = 0.0
      DO 200  L = 1,K
      READ(ICR,196) SYM(L), ALPHA2
196   FORMAT(F5.2,4X,3A4)
      LN = L + KTOTL
      DEPV = DEPV + C(LN) * SYM(L)
200   WRITE (LP,205 ) LN,C(LN), ALPHA2
205   FORMAT(1H ,I3,1X,E14.8, 5X, 3A4)
      WRITE (LP,210 ) DEPV, ALPHA1
210   FORMAT(21H DEPENDENT VARIABLE =,E14.8, 5X, 3A4)
      KTOTL = KTOTL + K
      IF(KTOTL - NR1) 180,215,215
215   SSQ = 0.0
      WRITE (LP,600) FMT
      WRITE (LP,220 )
220   FORMAT(1H0,3X,13HOBS. ACTIVITY,3X,14HCALC. ACTIVITY,9X, 3HDIF)
      SSQ1=0.0
      NL = 6
      DO 235  M=1,N
      READ (MT) V
      S=F
      DO 225 I = 1,NR1
225   S = S + C(I) * V(I)
      DIF = V(KNR) - S
      SSQ = DIF * DIF + SSQ
      WRITE (LP,230 ) V(KNR), S, DIF
      NL= NL + 1
      IF (NL - 54) 235,231,231
231   NL=0
      WRITE ( LP, 24)
230   FORMAT(1H ,3F17.7)
235   SSQ1 = V(KNR) * V(KNR) + SSQ1
      REWIND MT
      SSQ1 = SSQ1 - SUM(KNR) * SUM(KNR) * FN
C
C     DETERMINES SIGNIFICANCE OF DATA - F TEST
C     GIVES F VALUE
C
      TDF = FN - 1.0
      WRITE (LP,600) FMT
      WRITE (LP,237)
237   FORMAT (21HOSTATISTICAL ANALYSIS)
      WRITE (LP,240 )
240   FORMAT(20HOSOURCE OF VARIATION,6X,4HD.F.,7X,14HSUM OF SQUARES,
     17X,11HMEAN SQUARE)
      WRITE (LP,245 ) TDF,SSQ1
245   FORMAT (4X,5HTOTAL,F20.0,7X,E14.8)
      RSSQ = SSQ1 - SSQ
      FNR = FLOAT(KNR)
      DF2 = FN - FNR
      DF1 = TDF - DF2
      RMNSQ = RSSQ/DF1
      WRITE (LP,250 ) DF1,RSSQ,RMNSQ
```

```
250   FORMAT(4X,10HREGRESSION,F15.0,2(7X,E14.8))
      DMNSQ = SSQ/DF2
      WRITE (LP,255 ) DF2,SSQ,DMNSQ
255   FORMAT(4X,10HDEVIATIONS,F15.0,2(7X,E14.8))
      F = RMNSQ/DMNSQ
      WRITE (LP,260 ) F
260   FORMAT(4HOF =,F14.8)
C
C     DETERMINES COEFFICIENT OF MULTIPLE CORRELATION)
C
      R = SQRT(RSSQ/SSQ1)
      WRITE (LP,265 ) R
265   FORMAT(38HOCOEFFICIENT OF MULTIPLE CORRELATION =,F11.8)
C
C     DETERMINES EXPLAINED VARIANCE
C
      EV = 1.0 - (DMNSQ/(SSQ1/TDF))
      WRITE (LP,270 ) EV
270   FORMAT(31HOAMOUNT OF EXPLAINED VARIANCE =,F11.8/1HO)
C     DETERMINES T VALUE FOR EACH VARIABLE
      DO 275  I = 1, NR1
275   G(I) = C(I) / (SQRT(DMNSQ) * SQRT(DIAG(I)))
      WRITE (LP,280 ) DF2
280   FORMAT(31HOT VALUES FOR COEFFICIENTS WITH, F5.0,3H DF)
      WRITE (LP,285 ) (I,G(I), I=1,NR1)
285   FORMAT(3(3H T(,I3,3H) =, F14.8, 2X))
135   NRMX=NRMX-1
      IF (NRMX)1,290,1
290   CALL EXIT
      END
 END OF DATA
```

```
001
FREE WILSON ANALYSIS FOR ISOXAZOLO(3,4-D)PYRIMIDINES  12-20-71
DOSAGE REQUIRED TO PRODUCE A VIGOR OF 3 FOR INPUT
CROP IS CRAB GRASS  --  OMIT 23469, 23495, 25314
DEPENDENT VARIABLES ARE CH2CH3, CH3, N-O
 21 10
1.0                 1.0                 -20.00.50
-1.50-1.0 -0.75-1.0      1.0            1.0  0.25
1.0                      1.0            1.0  0.25
1.0                           1.0       1.0  1.0
     1.0            1.0                 1.0  0.25
          1.0                      1.0  1.0  0.25
-1.50-1.0 -0.75-1.0                1.0  1.0  0.25
1.0                                1.0  1.0  0.25
               1.0                 1.0  1.0  0.25
     1.0                      1.0       1.0  0.25
-1.50-1.0 -0.75-1.0           1.0       1.0  0.25
     1.0                           1.0  1.0  0.25
1.0                 1.0                 1.0  0.25
1.0                 -1.25-0.50-1.25-1.251.0  4.0
     1.0            -1.25-0.50-1.25-1.251.0  1.0
-1.50-1.0 -0.75-1.0 -1.25-0.50-1.25-1.251.0  2.0
               1.0  -1.25-0.50-1.25-1.251.0  8.0
               1.0            1.0       1.0  2.0
          1.0       1.0                 1.0  1.0
          1.0                 1.0       1.0  4.0
               1.0  1.0                 1.0  0.50
 4       A
-1.50    B
-1.0     C
-.75     D
-1.0     E
 4       F
-1.25    G
-.50     H
-1.25    I
-1.25    J
 1       K
-20.0    L
 END OF DATA
```

```
FREE WILSON ANALYSIS FOR ISOXAZOLO(3,4-D)PYRIMIDINES  12-20-71
DOSAGE REQUIRED TO PRODUCE A VIGOR OF 3 FOR INPUT
CROP IS CRAB GRASS  --  OMIT 23469, 23495, 25314
DEPENDENT VARIABLES ARE CH2CH3, CH3, N-O

INPUT DATA FOLLOWS

EQUATION    1     ACTIVITY =   0.500     INDEPENDENT VARIABLES FOLLOW
    1.000     0.0       0.0        0.0        1.000      0.0        0.0
    0.0     -20.000

EQUATION    2     ACTIVITY =   0.250     INDEPENDENT VARIABLES FOLLOW
   -1.500    -1.000    -0.750     -1.000      0.0        1.000      0.0
    0.0       1.000

EQUATION    3     ACTIVITY =   0.250     INDEPENDENT VARIABLES FOLLOW
    1.000     0.0       0.0        0.0        0.0        1.000      0.0
    0.0       1.000

EQUATION    4     ACTIVITY =   1.000     INDEPENDENT VARIABLES FOLLOW
    1.000     0.0       0.0        0.0        0.0        0.0        1.000
    0.0       1.000

EQUATION    5     ACTIVITY =   0.250     INDEPENDENT VARIABLES FOLLOW
    0.0       1.000     0.0        0.0        1.000      0.0        0.0
    0.0       1.000

EQUATION    6     ACTIVITY =   0.250     INDEPENDENT VARIABLES FOLLOW
    0.0       0.0       1.000      0.0        0.0        0.0        0.0
    1.000     1.000

EQUATION    7     ACTIVITY =   0.250     INDEPENDENT VARIABLES FOLLOW
   -1.500    -1.000    -0.750     -1.000      0.0        0.0        0.0
    1.000     1.000

EQUATION    8     ACTIVITY =   0.250     INDEPENDENT VARIABLES FOLLOW
    1.000     0.0       0.0        0.0        0.0        0.0        0.0
    1.000     1.000

EQUATION    9     ACTIVITY =   0.250     INDEPENDENT VARIABLES FOLLOW
    0.0       0.0       0.0        1.000      0.0        0.0        0.0
    1.000     1.000

EQUATION   10     ACTIVITY =   0.250     INDEPENDENT VARIABLES FOLLOW
    0.0       1.000     0.0        0.0        0.0        0.0        1.000
    0.0       1.000
```

```
EQUATION    11      ACTIV!TY =    0.250      INDEPENDENT VARIABLES FOLLOW
   -1.5CC     -1.CCC    -0.750    -1.000      0.0         0.0        1.0C0
    C.0        1.C00

EQUATION    12      ACTIVITY =    0.250      INDEPENDENT VARIABLES FOLLOW
    C.C        1.CC0     0.0        0.0       0.0         C.0        C.C
    1.CCC      1.CCC

EQUATION    13      ACTIVITY =    0.250      INDEPENDENT VARIABLES FOLLOW
    1.CCC      0.C       0.0        0.0       1.000       0.0        C.C
    C.C        1.CC0

EQUATION    14      ACTIVITY =    4.000      INDEPENDENT VARIABLES FOLLOW
    1.CC0      0.0       0.0        0.0      -1.250      -0.5C0     -1.250
   -1.25C      1.CC0

EQUATION    15      ACTIVITY =    1.000      INDEPENDENT VARIABLES FOLLOW
    C.0        1.CC0     0.0        0.0      -1.250      -0.500     -1.250
   -1.250      1.CC0

EQUATION    16      ACTIVITY =    2.000      INDEPENDENT VARIABLES FOLLOW
   -1.5CC     -1.CCC    -0.750    -1.000     -1.250      -0.500     -1.250
   -1.25C      1.CC0

EQUATION    17      ACTIVITY =    8.000      INDEPENDENT VARIABLES FOLLOW
    C.C        0.C       0.0        1.000    -1.250      -0.500     -1.25C
   -1.25C      1.CC0

EQUATION    18      ACTIVITY =    2.000      INDEPENDENT VARIABLES FOLLOW
    C.0        0.C       0.0        1.000     0.0         0.0        1.CCC
    C.C        1.CCC

EQUATION    19      ACTIVITY =    1.000      INDEPENDENT VARIABLES FOLLOW
    0.C        0.0       1.000      0.0       1.000       0.0        0.0
    C.0        1.C00

EQUATION    2C      ACTIVITY =    4.000      INDEPENDENT VARIABLES FOLLOW
    0.C        0.0       1.000      0.0       0.0         0.0        1.CC0
    0.0        1.000

EQUATION    21      ACTIVITY =    0.500      INDEPENDENT VARIABLES FOLLOW
    0.0        0.0       0.0        1.000     1.000       0.0        0.0
    0.0        1.000
```

```
FREE WILSON ANALYSIS FOR ISOXAZOLO(3,4-D)PYRIMIDINES  12-20-71
DOSAGE REQUIRED TO PRODUCE A VIGOR OF 3 FOR INPUT
CROP IS CRAB GRASS  --  OMIT 23469, 23495, 25314
DEPENDENT VARIABLES ARE CH2CH3, CH3, N-O

   21 COMPOUNDS        9 INDEPENDENT VARIABLES

VALUE OF THE DETERMINANT = 0.47541325E 09

REGRESSION CONSTANT =0.12738094E 01

SUBSTITUENT CONTRIBUTIONS

GROUP  1
  1 -.15196538E 00      B
  2 -.99676359E 00      C
  3 0.11534023E 01      D
  4 0.12532349E 01      E
DEPENDENT VARIABLE =-.89357519E 00      A

GROUP  2
  5 -.10660744E 01      G
  6 -.47882873E 00      H
  7 0.17553496E 00      I
  8 -.10744610E 01      J
DEPENDENT VARIABLE =0.26956635E 01      F

GROUP  3
  9 -.22211570E-01      L
DEPENDENT VARIABLE =0.44423139E 00      K
```

```
FREE WILSON ANALYSIS FOR ISOXAZOLO(3,4-D)PYRIMIDINES  12-20-71
DOSAGE REQUIRED TO PRODUCE A VIGOR OF 3 FOR INPUT
CROP IS CRAB GRASS  --  OMIT 23469, 23495, 25314
DEPENDENT VARIABLES ARE CH2CH3, CH3, N-O
```

OBS. ACTIVITY	CALC. ACTIVITY	DIF
0.5000000	0.5000004	-0.0000004
0.2500000	-0.1208075	0.3708075
0.2500000	0.6208030	-0.3708030
1.0000000	1.2751656	-0.2751656
0.2500000	-0.8112401	1.0612392
0.2500000	1.3305387	-1.0805387
0.2500000	-0.7164397	0.9664397
0.2500000	0.0251708	0.2248292
0.2500000	1.4303713	-1.1803713
0.2500000	0.4303692	-0.1803692
0.2500000	0.5335562	-0.2835562
0.2500000	-0.8196267	1.0696259
0.2500000	0.0335574	0.2164426
4.0000000	3.7952948	0.2047052
1.0000000	2.9504967	-1.9504967
2.0000000	3.0536842	-1.0536842
8.0000000	5.2004957	2.7995043
2.0000000	2.6803665	-0.6803665
1.0000000	1.3389254	-0.3389254
4.0000000	2.5805340	1.4194660
0.5000000	1.4387579	-0.9387579

```
FREE WILSON ANALYSIS FOR ISOXAZOLO(3,4-D)PYRIMIDINES  12-20-71
DOSAGE REQUIRED TO PRODUCE A VIGOR OF 3 FOR INPUT
CROP IS CRAB GRASS  --  OMIT 23469, 23495, 25314
DEPENDENT VARIABLES ARE CH2CH3, CH3, N-O

STATISTICAL ANALYSIS

SOURCE OF VARIATION      D.F.       SUM OF SQUARES        MEAN SQUARE
   TOTAL                 20.        0.74113113E 02
   REGRESSION             9.        0.51519196E 02       0.57243547E 01
   DEVIATIONS            11.        0.22593918E 02       0.20539923E 01

F =     2.78694057

COEFFICIENT OF MULTIPLE CORRELATION = 0.83375221

AMOUNT OF EXPLAINED VARIANCE = 0.44571418


T VALUES FOR COEFFICIENTS WITH  11. DF
T(  1) =   -0.28108257   T(  2) =   -1.50716400   T(  3) =    1.43389416
T(  4) =    1.89496231   T(  5) =   -1.67527294   T(  6) =   -0.45731235
T(  7) =    0.30960256   T(  8) =   -1.89509678   T(  9) =   -0.27208149
```

AUTHOR INDEX

SUBJECT INDEX